D0494642

Statistical Evidence in Medical Trials

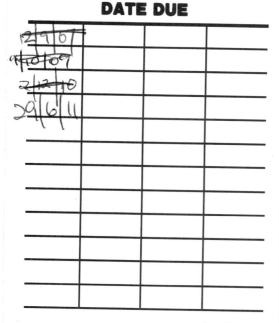

DATE DUE

2/9/07			
9/10/09			
2/12/10			
29/6/11			

Demco No. 62-0549

Statistical Evidence in Medical Trials

What Do the Data Really Tell Us?

Stephen D. Simon, Ph.D.

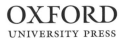

OXFORD

UNIVERSITY PRESS

OXFORD
UNIVERSITY PRESS

Great Clarendon Street, Oxford OX2 6DP

Oxford University Press is a department of the University of Oxford.
It furthers the University's objective of excellence in research, scholarship,
and education by publishing worldwide in

Oxford New York

Auckland Cape Town Dar es Salaam Hong Kong Karachi
Kuala Lumpur Madrid Melbourne Mexico City Nairobi
New Delhi Shanghai Taipei Toronto

With offices in

Argentina Austria Brazil Chile Czech Republic France Greece
Guatemala Hungary Italy Japan Poland Portugal Singapore
South Korea Switzerland Thailand Turkey Ukraine Vietnam

Oxford is a registered trade mark of Oxford University Press
in the UK and in certain other countries

Published in the United States
by Oxford University Press Inc., New York

British Library Cataloguing in Publication Data

Data available

Library of Congress Cataloging in Publication Data

Data available

Typeset by SPI Publisher Services, Pondicherry, India
Printed in Great Britain
on acid-free paper by
Biddles Ltd., King's Lynn, Norfolk

ISBN 0–19–856760–X   978–0–19–856760–8
ISBN 0–19–856761–8(Pbk.)   978–0–19–856761–5(Pbk.)

3 5 7 9 10 8 6 4 2

Contents

Preface

There is a story[1] about two doctors who are floating above the countryside in a hot-air balloon. They are drifting with the wind and enjoying the scenery, but after a couple of hours, they realize that they are totally lost. They see someone down on the ground, and shout down 'Hello! Can you tell us where we are?'

The person on the ground replies, 'you're fifty feet up in the air, in a hot-air balloon.'

One doctor turns to the other and says, 'That person on the ground must be a statistician.'

'How did you know?' came astonished reply from the ground.

'Only a statistician would provide an answer that was totally accurate and totally useless at the same time.'

In my stories, of course, the statistician always has the last word: 'Very good. But I can also tell that you two are doctors.'

It was the doctors' turn to be astonished. The statistician explained, 'Only a doctor would have such a good view of the area and still not have any idea where they were.'

If you are a doctor or any other health care professional, you have such a good view of the research. There are thousands of medical journals that publish hundreds of research articles each year. But with all that information, it is still difficult for you to know what is going on.

Several years ago, I became very interested in understanding how health care professionals made decisions. How did they choose which new therapies and treatments to adopt? When did the evidence in favor of a new practice become compelling enough to get them to drop an old and ingrained way of practicing their craft?

It is not an easy question to answer. Medical professionals who cling stubbornly to what they learned in school are not doing their job well. But adopting willy-nilly any new trend that comes along would make things even worse.

If you have ever agonized about whether to change your practice on the basis of a new research study, this book is for you. Is a research study definitive, or is it an interesting finding that needs replication? I can help answer this question. Not that I can better gauge the quality of the evidence,

---

[1] I cannot claim credit for this joke. It has been running around the Internet in various forms for years. Do a web search on the words 'joke hot-air balloon' for some examples.

but because I can help you ask the right questions. Was there a good control group? Did the researchers study the right patients? Did they measure the proper outcomes?

How did this all get started?

The original inspiration for this book came from the students in an informal class I was teaching at Children's Mercy Hospital in 1997. In a survey, I asked the students why they were taking the class. My hope was that this information would help me select future topics for discussion. A common response was along the lines of 'I want to understand the statistics used in medical journal articles.' So I prepared a talk called 'How to Read a Medical Journal Article.' I expanded the talk into a web page (www.childrens-mercy.org/stats/journal.asp).

Some of the original material that inspired this book can still be found there, as well as in a weblog that I started in 2004 (www.childrens-mercy.org/stats/weblog.asp).

Around the same time, I had the good fortune of being invited to write a series of articles about research for the Lab Corner section of the *Journal of Andrology*. This allowed me to further refine these ideas.

My other inspiration came from the invitations I got to participate in several journal clubs at Children's Mercy Hospital. The journal articles were always interesting and the discussions helped me polish the ideas that I am presenting here.

Outline of this book

The Introduction documents some of the weaknesses in published research of which you need to be aware. Some of you do not need any convincing that much of the research being published has serious limitations. This is where I make my case that you should worry more about how the data were collected rather than how it was analyzed. I also stress the importance of critical thinking.

'Apples or Oranges?' examines the quality of the control group. A carefully selected control group strengthen credibility of the research. If you want a technical term, this is often called the internal validity of the research.

'Who Was Left Out?' considers exclusions before the study started, and exclusions during the study. If important segments of the population are left out, you may have difficulty generalizing the results of the study. This is often called the external validity of the research.

'Mountain or Molehill?' examines the clinical relevance of the outcome. The outcome measure has to be properly collected and has to measure something of interest to your patients. The size of the study has to be large enough to produce reasonably precise estimates and the difference between the treatment and control group has to be large enough to have a clinical impact.

'What Do the Other Witnesses Say?' discusses how to look at additional corroborating evidence outside the journal article itself. Corroborating evidence is especially important for observational studies, because it is rare that a single observational study provides definitive results entirely by itself. Rather, it is a collection of observational studies, all looking at the problem from a different perspective, that can provide persuasive evidence. This section is loosely based on the nine factors to assess a causal relationship that Sir Bradford Hill developed in 1966.

'Do the Pieces Fit Together?' applies the same principles of statistical evidence to meta-analyses and systematic overviews. Study heterogeneity, study quality, and publication bias are serious threats to the validity of a systematic overview.

'What Do All These Numbers Mean?' gives a nontechnical explanation for some of the statistics used in hypothesis testing, such as p-values and confidence intervals. It also explains the various measures of risk, like the odds ratio, relative risk, and number needed to treat.

'Where Is the Evidence?' gives a brief overview of how to search for research articles. The first step is to structure your question carefully. Then you should start with high-level sources first, sources that include summaries and systematic overviews. These are better than using PubMed or the Internet, which often offer too much information for you to synthesize properly. If you do need to use PubMed or the Internet, though, I offer some tips for refining your search.

Who is this book for?

I am writing this book for any health care professional who is making the effort to read and evaluate medical publications. Do you update and modify your clinical practice on the basis of what you read in the research journals? I have guidelines that can help you.

Nonmedical professionals can also benefit from this book. I do use a few technical medical terms, but as long as words like 'myocardial infarction' do not give you a heart attack, you will be just fine. Indeed, many people like me who do not have specialized medical training will still read medical journals. Journalists, for example, have to write about the peer-reviewed literature for the public and they need to know when researchers are over-hyping their research findings. Lawyers involved with malpractice suits need to understand which medical practices have been supported by medical research, which practices have been discredited, and which practices still require additional research. More and more patients want to research their own diseases so they can discuss treatment options intelligently with their doctors.

And while I focus mostly on medical examples, the general principles apply to other areas as well. If you work in a nonmedical field, but you read peer-reviewed journals and try to incorporate their findings into your job, my guidelines can help you.

I did not write this book to teach you how to conduct good research. I wrote it for *consumers* of research, not producers of research. Even so, when you plan your research you should try to use a research design that is most likely to be persuasive. To that extent, my book can help.

There are several things I am quite proud of in this book:

Extensive use of real world examples. There are a lot of fascinating research papers out there, and they tell an intriguing story. These papers pose interesting questions like 'what sort of person would volunteer to have a spinal tap done as part of a research study' and 'why would a doctor flip a sterilized coin in the operating room?' I have included hundreds of citations in this book, and many of these examples have the full text on the web for free.

Focus on statistics issues. When you are trying to assess the quality of a medical publication, most of the issues touch directly on Statistics. And yet, Statistics is the one area that medical professionals are intimidated by. Well, Statistics is not brain surgery, and you are capable of understanding the concepts.

Avoidance of formulas and technical language. People think that Statistics is a bunch of numbers and formulas, but there are a lot of nonquantitative issues in how statistics are applied in research. When you are trying to assess the credibility of a research study, these nonquantitative concerns are far more important than any formulas or statistical calculations.

Presentation of counterpoints. While I am a big fan of randomization intention to treat analysis and so forth, these approaches can be overrated. By presenting counter-arguments that these approaches are not all they are cracked up to be, I hope to bring to life some of the on-going controversies in Evidence-Based Medicine.

On Your Own Exercises. There is great value in applying the skills you have just learned, and I offer some practice exercises at the end of most chapters. These exercises use abstracts and excerpts from open source journals. You can find answers to the exercises at my web site (www.childrensmercy.org/stats/evidence/answers.asp).

Acknowledgments

I could not have written this book without the hard work of my administrative assistant, Linda Foland, who has tamed a massive database of almost 5,000 bibliographic entries. She has also applied her sharp editorial eye to the web pages that eventually morphed into this book that you are now reading. Linda was preceded by two other very capable administrative assistants, Carla Liebentritt and Meg Goodloe, who have deservedly gone on to bigger and better things, but who were of immense help while I had the privilege of working with them.

It has been great to work with Alison Jones at Oxford University Press. She has patiently guided me along the process, and has tolerated many slipped deadlines.

All of the 'On Your Own' exercises as well as the graphs and figures that you see in this book come from papers published by Biomed Central under the open access license. This license allows you flexibility to use to copy and display the work or any derivative work as long as you cite the original source. I have to thank the authors who are brave enough to try this publication model, as it makes it so much easier to produce my web pages and this book.

I also have learned a lot from the participants of various Internet email discussion groups (especially edstat-l, epidemio-l, evidence-based-health, irbforum, and stat-l), who have shared their wisdom with me and the rest of world. My meager contributions to these groups can only be a small and partial repayment for all the things that I have learned.

Thanks also go to the doctors, nurses, and other health-care professionals at Children's Mercy Hospital, who helped keep me on my toes by asking difficult questions that forced me to think hard about the process of research. Because of you, my job is a constant intellectual challenge.

Most of all, I have to thank my wife, Cathy, who has always provided support and encouragement throughout the entire process. Cathy, your unwavering belief in me gave me the spark to persevere.

Overview

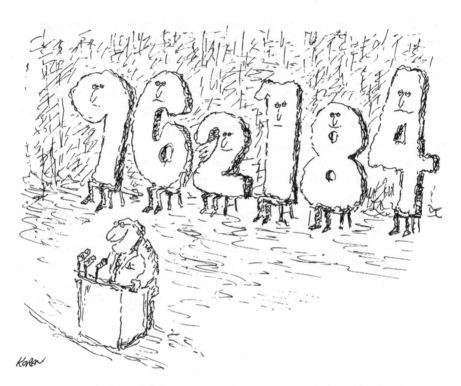

"Tonight, we're going to let the statistics speak for themselves."

There is an enormous mistrust of statistics in the real world. To the extent that it makes people skeptical, that's good. To the extent it turns them cynical, that's bad. There is a viewpoint, championed by too many people, that all statistics are worthless. I call this viewpoint statistical nihilism. Here is an instructive example:

> The paradigm of evidence-based medicine now being proposed is nothing but the thinly disguised worship of statistical methods and techniques. The value and worth of nearly all medications of proven effectiveness were developed without the benefits of statistical tools, to wit, digitalis, colchicine, aspirin, penicillin, and so on. Statistical analyses only demonstrate levels of numeric association or, at best,

> impart a numeric dimension to the level of confidence—or lack thereof—that chance contributed to the shape and distribution of the data set under consideration. Statistical association cannot replace causal relation—which, in the final analysis, is the bedrock on which good medical practice must rest. (Boba 1998)

There are a lot more examples out there. Usually, people who adopt statistical nihilism have an axe to grind. In their minds, there is a problem with most of the research in a certain area, and rather than attack the research directly, they try to undermine the research by citing all the flaws in the statistical methodology. Of course, you can always find flaws in any research including in the statistical methodology. The perfect statistical analysis has yet to be performed.

What is missing among these statistical nihilists is a sense of proportion. Some statistical flaws are so serious as to invalidate the research. Other flaws raise enough concern that you should demand additional corroborating evidence (such as replication of the study). Other flaws are mere trifles.

If you are a nihilist, life is easy. Just keep a list of statistical flaws handy and one of them is bound to apply to the research study that you dislike.

The real world, of course, is much more complex. Medical care givers do indeed change their practices in response to the publication of well-designed research studies. These changes follow extensive debate and careful review of all the evidence[1].

Research has also shown that adults who take a daily dose of aspirin can reduce their risk of heart attacks and strokes (Physicians' Health Study Research Group 1989). The Women's Health Initiative published findings (Rossouw 2002) that indicated that hormone replacement therapy in post-menopausal women may actually be harmful rather than helpful. This followed a couple of other studies (Hulley 1998; Herrington 2000) that laid the seeds of doubt about this practice. Another spectacular failure that was discovered through careful research was that drugs that suppress cardiac arryhtmias may actually increase mortality (Epstein 1993).

On the other hand, it helps to recognize and be constantly vigilant for the many limitations in medical research. A large number of review articles have demonstrated that the publications in many medical disciplines have serious limitations and leave much room for improvement. One of the best examples is a large-scale review by Ben Thornley and Clive Adams of research on schizophrenia (Thornley 1998). You can find the full text at: www.bmj.com/cgi/content/full/317/7167/1181 and it is well worth reading. Thornley and Adams looked at the quality of clinical trials for treating schizophrenia. Since they work for the Cochrane Collaboration Group that

---

[1] The following examples are drawn mostly from a website that Benjamin Djulbegovic developed on randomized trials that changed medical practice based on comments he received on the Evidence-Based Health email discussion group. You can find even more good examples at www.hsc.usf.edu/bdjulbeg/oncology/RCT-practice-change.htm.

provides systematic reviews of the results of medical trials, they are in a good position to write such an article.

Thornley and Adams actually identified over 2,500 studies of schizophrenia, but decided to summarize only the first 2,000 that they uncovered. Perhaps they reached the point of sheer exhaustion. I am very impressed at the amount of work this must have taken.

The research covered 50 years, starting in 1948 through 1997. The research covered a variety of therapies: drug therapies, psychotherapy, policy or care packages, or physical interventions like electroconvulsive therapy.

What did Thornley and Adams find? It was not a pretty picture. First, researchers in schizophrenia studied the wrong patients. Most studies used institutionalized patients, who are easier to recruit and follow up with, but who do not provide a good representation of all the patients with schizophrenia. Readers would probably be interested as much in community-based studies, if not more interested, but only 14% of the studies were community based. From the perspective of the researchers, of course, it is a whole lot easier to use institutionalized patients, because if they do not show up for their six-month evaluation, you know where to find them.

Second, the researchers also did not study enough patients. Thornley and Adams estimated that a good study of schizophrenia should have at least 300 patients in each group. This would be based on rates of improvements that might be expected for an active drug compared to placebo effects. Even though the desired sample size was 300, it turns out that the average study had only 65. Only 3% of the studies had 300 or more patients. From the perspective of researchers, it is a whole lot easier to study a small number of patients because you can finish the publication with less effort and money.

Third, the researchers did not study the patients long enough. A good study of schizophrenia should last for six months or more; long-term changes are more important than short-term changes. Unfortunately, more than half of the studies lasted for six weeks or less. From the perspective of the researchers, it is a whole lot easier to focus on short-term outcomes because you can finish the study a lot faster.

Finally, the researchers did not measure these patients consistently. In the 2,000 studies, the researchers used 640 ways to measure the impact of the interventions. Granted, there are a lot of dimensions to schizophrenia and there were measures of symptoms, behavior, cognitive functioning, side effects, social functioning, and so forth. Still, there is no justification for using so many different measurements. Imagine how hard this makes it for anyone to summarize the results of this research. Failure to use and re-use a few standardized assessments has led to a very fragmentary (dare I say, schizophrenic) picture about schizophrenia treatments.

Like all the previous problems, this can be explained from the perspective of convenience. It is a whole lot easier to develop your own outcome measure than to try to adapt somebody else's.

This publication suggests that a big problem with medical research is that the researchers have a strong tendency to conduct research that is easy to do. The research that is relevant to practicing clinicians is much harder. This is hardly surprising. Research on schizophrenia is especially hard to do well. Can you imagine trying to discuss an informed consent document with a patient who suffers from schizophrenia?

I do not want this example to turn you into a statistical nihilist, though. The take-home message from Thornley and Adams is that just because the research is peer-reviewed does not mean that it is perfect. I hope it helps you identify factors that limit the quality of peer-reviewed research.

If you practice medicine intelligently, you have to incorporate some research studies into your clinical practice and disregard other studies. Which studies do you incorporate? It depends on the quality of evidence in the article. Was there a good comparison group? How were dropouts and exclusions handled? Did they measure the outcome variable well? What other corroborating evidence is there? Those are questions that I will address in the rest of the book.

1 Apples or Oranges? Selection of the Control Group

1.1 Introduction

Almost all research involves comparison. Do women who take Tamoxifen have a lower rate of breast cancer recurrence than women who take a placebo? Do left-handed people die at an earlier age than right-handed people? Are men with severe vertex balding more likely to develop heart disease than men with no balding?

In each of these situations, you are making a comparison between a control group and a treatment/exposure group. I will use the terms treatment and exposure interchangably throughout this book, though I will reserve treatment for those conditions which represent an effort to produce a beneficial result and exposure to represent a condition that is potentially harmful. You would call drinking water from a natural spring a treatment, but drinking water from a contaminated well an exposure. The distinction between treatment and exposure is not that critical though, and when I discuss a generic 'treatment' in this book, feel free to substitute the word "exposure" and vice versa.

When you make such a comparison between a treatment group and a control group, you want a *fair comparison*. You want the control group to be identical to the treatment group in all respects, except for the treatment in question. You want an apples-to-apples comparison.

1.1.1 Covariate imbalance

Sometimes, however, you get an unfair comparison, an apples-to-oranges comparison. The control group differs on some important characteristics that might influence the outcome measure. This is known as covariate imbalance. Covariate imbalance is not an insurmountable problem, but it does make a study less authoritative.

Women who take oral contraceptives appear to have a higher risk of cervical cancer. But covariate imbalance might be producing an artificial rise in cancer rates for this group. Women who take oral contraceptives behave, as a group, differently than other women. For example, women who take oral contraceptives have a larger number of Pap smears. This is probably because these women visit their doctors more regularly in order to get their prescriptions refilled and therefore have more opportunities to be offered a Pap smear. This difference could lead to an increase in the number of detected cancer cases. Perhaps the other women have just as much cancer, but it is more likely to remain undetected.

There are many other variables that influence the development of cervical cancer: age of first intercourse, number of sexual partners, use of condoms, and smoking habits. If women who take oral contraceptives differ in any of these lifestyle factors, then that might also produce a difference in cervical cancer rates.[1]

1.1.2   Case study: vitamin C and cancer

Paul Rosenbaum, in the first chapter of his book, *Observational Studies*, gives a fascinating example of an apples-to-oranges comparison. Ewan Cameron and Linus Pauling published an observational study of Vitamin C as a treatment for advanced cancer (Cameron 1976). For each patient, ten matched controls were selected with the same age, gender, cancer site, and histological tumor type. Patients receiving vitamin C survived four times longer than the controls ($p < 0.0001$).

Cameron and Pauling minimize the lack of randomization:

> Even though no formal process of randomization was carried out in the selection of our two groups, we believe that they come close to representing random subpopulations of the population of terminal cancer patients in the Vale of Leven Hospital.

Ten years later, the Mayo Clinic conducted a randomized experiment which showed no statistically significant effect of vitamin C (Moertel 1985). Why did the Cameron and Pauling study differ from the Mayo study?

The first limitation of the Cameron and Pauling study was that all of their patients received vitamin C and followed prospectively. The control group represented a retrospective chart review. You should be cautious about any comparison of prospective data to retrospective data.

But there was a more important issue. The treatment group represented patients newly diagnosed with terminal cancer. The control group was selected from death certificate records. So this was clearly an apples-to-oranges comparison because the initial prognosis was worse in the control group than in the treatment group. As Rosenbaum says so well: '*one can say with total confidence, without reservation or caveat, that the prognosis of the patient who is already dead is not good*' (p. 4).

---

[1] The possibility that oral contraceptives causes an increase in the risk of cervical cancer is quite complex; a good summary of all the issues involved is available at: www.jhuccp.org/pr/a9/a9chap5.shtml.

The prognosis of a patient with a diagnosis of terminal cancer is also not good, but at least a few of these patients will be misdiagnosed. The ones in the control group, the ones that entered the study clutching their death certificates, had no misdiagnosis.

1.1.3   Apples or oranges? What to look for

When the treatment group is apples and the control group is oranges, you cannot make a fair comparison. To ensure that the researchers made an apples-to-apples comparison, ask the following questions:

Did the authors use randomization? In some studies, the researchers control who gets the new therapy and who gets the standard (control) therapy. When the researchers have this level of control, they almost always will randomize the choice. This type of study, a randomized study, is a very effective and very simple way to prevent covariate imbalance.

If randomization was not done, how were the patients selected? Several alternative approaches are available when the researchers have control of treatment assignment, but minimization is the only credible alternative. When researchers do not have control over treatment assignments, you have an observational study. The three major observational studies, cohort designs, case-control designs, and historical controls, all have weaknesses, but may represent the best available approach that is practical and ethical.

Did the authors use matching to prevent covariate imbalance? Matching is a method for selecting subjects that ensures a similar set of patients for the control group. A crossover design represents the ideal form of matching because each subject serves as his or her own control. Stratification ensures that broad demographic groups are equally represented in the treatment and control group.

Did the authors use statistical adjustments to control for covariate imbalance? Covariate adjustment uses statistical methods to try to correct for any existing imbalance. These methods work well, but only on variables that can be measured easily and accurately.

1.2   Randomly selected controls

Randomization is the assignment of treatment groups through the use of a random device, like the flip of a coin or the roll of a die, or numbers randomly generated by a computer. Randomization is not always possible, practical, or ethical. But when you can use randomization, it greatly adds to the credibility of the research study.

Example: In a study of treatments for osteoarthritis of the knee (Teeka-chunhatean 2004), 200 patients suffering from osteoarthritis of the knee were randomly assigned to receive either DJW (Duhuo Jisheng Wan, a Chinese herbal remedy) and a placebo for diclofenac or diclofenac and a placebo for DJW. Patients were evaluated on visual analog scale (VAS) score that assessed pain and stiffness, Lequesne's functional index, time for climbing up ten steps, as well as physician's and patients' overall opinions on improvement.

Example: In a study of critical appraisal skills training (Taylor 2004), 145 health professionals were randomly assigned to either receive immediate training in a half-day critical appraisal skills workshop or were placed on a waiting list for a future workshop. These subjects were evaluated on knowledge attitudes and behaviors relating to evidence-based medicine.

In both studies the researchers decided who got what. This is a hallmark of a randomized design and it only can occur when the patients and/or their doctors have no say in the assignment. This is an incredible gift that patients in a research study offer you. They sacrifice their ability to choose among two or more therapies and instead let that choice be decided by the flip of a coin.

1.2.1   How does randomization help?

Randomization helps ensure that both measurable and immeasurable factors are balanced out across both the standard and the new therapy, assuring a fair comparison. Used correctly, it also guarantees that no conscious or subconscious efforts were used to allocate subjects in a biased way.

There are situations where covariate imbalance can appear, even in a well-randomized study (Roberts 1999). Just as you have no guarantee that a flip of 100 coins will yield exactly 50 heads and 50 tails, you have no guarantee that covariate imbalances cannot creep into a randomized study once in a while. This is not just a theoretical concern. One article (Mann 2002) argues that a difference in baseline stroke severity in a randomized trial of tPA produced an incorrect assertion of the effectiveness of this treatment.

Randomization relies on the law of large numbers. With small sample sizes, covariate imbalance may still sneak in. A study examining the probability of covariate imbalance (Hsu 1989) showed that total sample sizes less than 10 could have a 50% chance or higher of having a categorical covariate with levels twice as large in one group than the other. This study also showed that total sample sizes of 40 or greater would have very little chance of such a serious imbalance, and a total of 20–40 subjects would be acceptable if there were only one or two important covariates.

1.2.2   A fishy story about randomization

I was told this story but have no way of verifying its accuracy. It is one of those stories that if it is not true, it should be. A long, long, time ago, a research group wanted to examine a pollutant to find concentration levels that would kill fish. This research required that 100 fish be separated into five tanks, each of which would get a different level of the pollutant. The researchers caught the first 20 fish and put them in the first tank, then put the next 20 fish in a second tank, and so forth. The last 20 fish went into the fifth tank. Each fish tank got a different concentration of the pollutant. When the research was done, the mortality was related not to the dosage, but to the order in which the tanks were filled, with the worst outcomes being in the first tank filled and the best outcomes in the last tank filled. What happened was that the slow-moving, easy-to-catch fish (the weakest and most sickly) were all allocated to the first tank. The fast-moving, hard-to-catch fish (the strongest and healthiest) ended up in the last tank.

Failure to randomize in this study ruined the entire effort. The huge imbalance caused by putting the sickest fish in the first tank and the healthiest fish in the last tank overwhelmed any differences in mortality caused by varying levels of the pollutant.

1.2.3   The mechanics of randomization

Random assignment means that the choice is left to some device that is inherently random and unpredictable. A flip of a coin is one approach, but usually a table of random numbers or a random number generator is more practical. I cannot think of anything more boring than flipping a coin 200 times.

Table 1.1 illustrates the simplest way to randomize an experiment. The trick is to recognize that sorting by a column of random numbers puts the data in a random order.

You can apply this trick to other situations where randomization is needed. Suppose, for example, that you have a list of 100 patients and

Table 1.1.   A simple approach to produce a randomization list.

Step 1. Arrange your data in a systematic order.	Step 2. Attach a column of random numbers.	Step 3. Sort by the column of random numbers.
T	T 0.608	C 0.016
C	C 0.739	C 0.030
T	T 0.831	T 0.608
C	C 0.016	C 0.739
T	T 0.759	T 0.759
C	C 0.877	T 0.830
T	T 0.830	T 0.831
C	C 0.030	C 0.877

you want to select 25 of them and send them each a survey. Just list the patients in alphabetical order. Attach a random number to each patients's name. Then sort the patient list by the random number. This puts the patient names in a random order, and you select the first 25 names on the list. If one of the patients turns out to be ineligible, then just go to the 26th name on the list.

Often, researchers will use block randomization. This approach creates randomization within small blocks, usually every 6 to 10 patients. This guarantees that your list will retain exact balance at the end of each block and will only show small degrees of imbalance in-between. In contrast, randomization across an entire very long list will show some random drift which would lead to serious imbalances partway through the study. If the experiment ends early, block randomization will ensure a greater degree of balance than simple randomization.

1.2.4 Concealing the randomization list

Another important aspect of randomization is concealed allocation, which is withholding the randomization list from those involved with recruiting subjects. This concealment occurs until after subjects agree to participate and the recruiter determines that the patient is eligible for the study. Only then is a sealed envelope opened that reveals the treatment status. Concealed allocation can also be done through a special phone number that the doctor calls to discover the treatment status.

Please note that concealing the randomization list is not the same as blinding the study (a topic I discuss later in this book). Certain treatments, such as surgery, cannot be blinded, but the allocation list can still be concealed. Consider, for example, a randomized trial comparing laparoscopic surgery to traditional surgery. After the fact, the patient can tell by the size of the scar what type of surgery they received. But the choice as to what type of surgery that the patient receives could be made as the patient is being sedated. There is an example of a research study where a sterilized coin was flipped in the operating room to decide which surgery will be used (Hollis 1999).

If the randomization list is not concealed, doctors have the ability to consciously or unconsciously influence the composition of the groups. They can do this by applying exclusion criteria differentially or by delaying entry of a certain healthier (or unhealthier) subject so he/she gets into the 'desirable' group. Unblinded allocation schemes tend, on average to overstate the effectiveness of the new therapy 30–40% (Schulz 1996).

There are many stories of physicians who have tried and succeeded in recruiting a patient into a preferred group. If the treatment allocation is hidden in sealed envelopes, they can hold it up to a strong light. If the sealed envelopes are not sequentially numbered, they can open several envelopes at once. If the allocation is controlled by a central operator, they can call and ask for the allocation of several patients at once.

When a doctor has an overt preference to enroll a patient into one group over another, it raises ethical issues and perhaps the doctor should not be participating in the trial. You should only participate in a research study if you believe there is genuine uncertainty about whether the new therapy or the standard therapy is better. If not, you have no business participating in a study where some of your patients will be randomized to a treatment that you consider inferior. Unfortunately, some doctors will continue to participate in these trials but will try to skew the enrollment of some or all of the patients towards a favored therapy.

Concealed allocation only makes sense for a truly randomized study. If patients are assigned in an alternating fashion, concealed allocation is like buying a fancy burglar alarm and leaving the front door wide open. As you will see in the next section, alternating assignments is a bad idea, but it is even worse because the doctors will immediately recognize where the next patient is going to be allocated. This makes it easy for them to recruit preferentially to a specific treatment if they wish.

1.2.5 Ethical and practical constraints on randomization

There are many situations where randomization is not practical or possible. Sometimes patients have a strong preference for one particular treatment and would not consider the possibility of being randomized into a different treatment. Surgery is one area with strong patient preferences especially for newer approaches like laparoscopic surgery (Lefering 2003).

Randomization is also problematic for interventions that are already known to be effective. While further research would help better define these advantages, you cannot ask half of your patients to sacrifice the benefits of the new intervention. A good example of this is breastfeeding, which has a whole host of positive effects.[2] There is still ongoing research to identify and better quantify these and other benefits, but almost none of this research is randomized (Kramer 2002 is a notable exception). Some nonrandomized studies of the relationship between breastfeeding and intelligence have failed to account for the fact that the breastfeeding mothers tend to be better educated, have higher socioeconomic status and that their babies tend to grow up in an environment that has greater overall levels of stimulation (Jain 2002). Still, it would be unethical to ask a random half of new mothers to sacrifice the benefits of breastfeeding. While this sometimes leads to limitations on what you can infer from these studies, that is the price you pay to live in an ethical society.

Randomization also does not work when you are studying noxious agents, like second-hand cigarette smoke or noisy workplaces. It would be unethical to deliberately expose people to any of these agents, so we have

---

[2] A nice summary of these benefits is available at: www.breastfeeding.com/all_about/all_about_more.html.

to collect data on those people who are unavoidably exposed to these things.

Sometimes, the sample sizes required or the duration of the study make it difficult to use randomization. Diseases like cancer that have a long latency period are especially hard to study with a randomized design.

Retrospective studies, where the outcome of interest has already occurred and/or you are looking at factors in the past that might have caused this outcome, are also impossible to randomize, unless you have a time machine. (See Leibovici 2001 for an amusing exception to this rule, though.)

Sometimes, the groups being studied existed before the start of the research. Genetic conditions like Down's syndrome cannot be randomly assigned to half of the patients in your study. I like to think of these situations as cases where God does the randomization.

Sometimes researchers just do not want to go to the effort of randomizing. If you assign the treatment or therapy, rather than letting the patients and their doctors choose, you have to expend a lot of energy. Is it worth the effort? It is usually faster and cheaper to use existing nonrandomized databases. You get a lot larger sample size for your money. Depending on the situation, that might be enough to counterbalance the advantages of randomization.

A nonrandomized study might also be a useful prelude in the planning of an expensive randomized trial. The nonrandomized trial would help you better understand and prepare for the resource requirements and familiarize your staff with the mechanics of treating and evaluating your research subjects.

1.2.6   Randomization: What to look for

If a study is randomized, look for the following features:

- Was there a description of the source of randomness? Did the researchers use a table of random numbers? Did they use a computer to generate random numbers?
- Did the researchers conceal the randomization list from the doctors during the recruitment of patients?

1.3   Variations on randomization

There are three variations to randomization where the researchers have control over treatment assignment, but they use something other than a table of random numbers for the assignment. The first approach, minimization, is a credible and reasonable choice, but the other two approaches, alternating assignment and haphazard assignment, do not have much to recommend them.

1.3.1 Minimization

An alternative, when the researchers have sufficient control, is to allocate the assignments so that at each step, the covariate imbalance is minimized. So if the treatment group has a slight surplus of older patients and the next patient to join the study is also older than average, then that patient would be assigned to the control group so as to reduce the age discrepancy.

Example: In a study of behavioral counseling (Steptoe 1999), twenty general practices were allocated either to use behavioral counseling based on the stages of change model for all their patients, or no counseling other than what their current standard of care. These practices were assigned using minimization to ensure balance on three factors: the degree of under-privileged patients being served, the patient to nurse ratio of the practice, and fund holding status.

Minimization is a good approach if there are one or two covariates which are especially important and which are easily measured at the start of the study. It will perform better than randomization on those factors, although there is no guarantee of covariate balance for other covariates not used in the minimization. Minimization also cannot control for unmeasured co-variates.

There is more effort required in setting up a study with minimization. You need a computer to be available at the time and location of the recruitment of each patient because you cannot just print a list ahead of time. Another difficulty is that minimization is open to possible abuse because doctors might be able to predict what the next assignment would be.

1.3.2 Alternating assignment

Another approach used in place of randomization is to alternate the assignment, so that every even patient is in the treatment group and every odd patient is in the control group. Alternating assignment was popular in trials before World War II; it was felt that researchers would not understand and not tolerate randomization (Yoshioka 1998).

Example: In a study of patients with cystic fibrosis (Homnick 1999), the first patient was randomly assigned either manual chest physiotherapy, or a flutter device to treat acute pulmonary exacerbation. After the first patient, each additional patient was assigned to the alternate approach.

Example: In a study of patients with penetrating eye injuries (Lakits 1998), patients were assigned alternately to either helical computed tomography or conventional computed tomography. Images were assessed for the ability to detect and accurately localize foreign bodies.

Alternating assignment seems on the surface to be a good approach, but it can sometimes lead to trouble. This is especially true when one patient has a direct or indirect influence on the next patient. You may have seen this level of influence if you grow vegetables in a garden. If you have a row of cabbages, for example, you will often see a pattern of big cabbage, little cabbage, big cabbage, little cabbage, etc. What happens, if the cabbages are planted a bit too closely, is that one of the cabbages will grow just a bit faster at first. It will extend into the neighboring cabbage's territory, stealing some of the nutrients and water, and thus growing even faster at the expense of the neighbor. If you had assigned a fertilizer to every other cabbage, you would probably see an artificial difference because of the alternating pattern in growth within a row.

This alternating pattern can also occur in medicine. Consider, for example, a study of how much time doctors spend with their patients. If the first patient takes longer than expected, the doctor will probably rush a bit with the second patient in order to keep from falling further behind schedule. On the other hand, if the first patient finishes quickly, then the doctor will feel more relaxed and might tend to take a bit more time with the next patient.

In some situations, alternating assignment would be tolerable, but there is no good reason to prefer this over random assignment. You should be skeptical of this approach because studies with alternating assignment will tend, on average, to overstate the effectiveness of a new therapy by 15% (Colditz 1989).

1.3.3   Haphazard assignment

Another choice that researchers will make is to base assignments on some arbitrary value. Often it is the evenness/oddness of the arbitrary number that determines the treatment assignment. For example, patients born on even-numbered dates would be assigned to the treatment group and those born on odd-numbered dates would be assigned to the control group. Some months have more odd days than even days (actually my life seems to have more than its fair share of odd days). This is a nitpick, but, more importantly, an arbitrary or haphazard number is never going to be as good as a purely random number. The haphazard assignment will always cast a shadow of doubt over the research study. This is a shame, because almost every study with haphazard assignment could have been run as a randomized study with just a little more fuss.

Example: In a study of heparinized saline to maintain the patency of patient catheters (Kulkarni 1994), patients admitted on odd-numbered dates received heparinized saline and patients admitted on even-numbered dates received normal saline.

Example: In a study of supplemental oxygen treatment for the treatment of stroke (Ronning 1999), patients born on even days were assigned to the supplemental oxygen group and patients born on odd days were assigned to the control group.

Example: In a study of interview methods for measuring risk behavior in injecting drug users (Des Jarlais 1999), patients were assigned either to a face-to-face interview or to audio-computer-assisted self-interviewing, depending on which week it was. The interview approach alternated from week to week. The patients were assessed to see if reporting of HIV risk behaviors changes between the interview methods.

In some situations, haphazard assignment might be tolerable, but there is no good reason to use this approach. The first study mentioned above was excluded from a meta-analysis of heparinized saline (Randolph 1998) because the reviewers felt the quality level was too low.

1.3.4   Variations on randomized studies: What to look for

When a study was not randomized, look for the following features:
For a study using minimization:

- Which covariates were used to assess balance?
- Were any important covariates ignored?

For studies using alternating assignments or haphazard assignments:

- Did the authors provide a justification for this approach?
- What possible artificial patterns in the assignments might create an artefactual relationship with the treatment assignment?

1.4   Nonrandomized studies

As mentioned earlier, there are many situations where randomization is not ethical, practical, or possible. Sometimes, researchers could not in good conscience assign a dangerous exposure randomly to half of their patients. Sometimes researchers do not have the resources to randomize patients. Sometimes patients and/or their physicians will select which therapy they receive. Sometimes the treatment or exposure variable represents a group that existed before the start of the research.

In these situations where randomization is not possible, you are looking at an observational study. There are four major flavors of observational studies: cohort studies, case-control studies, cross-sectional studies, and historical-control studies.

1.4.1   The cohort study

In a cohort study, a group of patients has a certain exposure or condition. They are compared to a group of patients without that exposure or condition. Does the exposed cohort differ from the unexposed cohort on an outcome of interest?

Example: In a study of suicide among Swedish men in the Swedish military service conscription register (Gunnell 2005), 987,308 men registered between 1968 and 1994 were divided into nine groups on the basis of four intelligence tests. These men were also linked to a Swedish cause of death register which identified a total of 2,811 suicides among these men. For each of the four intelligence tests, men scoring lower tended to have a higher rate of suicide.

Example: In a study of psychotic symptoms in young people (Henquet 2005), a sample of young adults aged 14–24 years were divided into a group of 320 with admitted use of cannabis and a group of 2,117 did not admit to cannabis use. Both groups were followed four years later for psychotic symptoms.

Cohort studies are intuitively appealing and selection of a control group is usually not too difficult. You have to be very wary of covariate imbalance, but other observational designs are likely to have even more problems. Do not worry about every possible covariate imbalance. You should look for large imbalances, especially for covariates which are closely related to the outcome variable.

When you are studying a very rare outcome, the sample size may have to be extremely large. As a rough rule of thumb, you need to observe 25–50 outcomes in each group in order to have a reasonable level of precision. So when a condition occurs only once in every thousand patients, a cohort study would require tens of thousands of patients.

You want to avoid 'leaky groups' in a cohort design. If the exposure group includes some unexposed patients and the control group includes some exposed patients, then any effect you are trying to detect will be diluted. Be especially aware of situations where one group is more leaky than the other.

For example, many studies will classify people into various levels of caffeine exposure on the basis of how much coffee they drink. Although coffee is the major source of caffeine for most people, failure to ask about other sources of caffeine consumption can lead to serious errors. A rabid Diet Coke drinker might mistakenly be classified into the low-caffeine consumption group (Brown 2001).

Dietary studies will sometimes rely on household food surveys, but these need adjustment for the varying consumption of individual family members. For example, within the same family, males (especially boys aged 11–17 years) will have higher average intakes of calories and nutrients (Nelson 1986).

1.4.2   The case-control study

A case-control study selects patients on the basis of an outcome, such as development of breast cancer, and are compared to a group of patients without that outcome. Do the cases differ from the controls in some exposures?

Example: In a study of asthma deaths (Anderson 2005), researchers selected 532 patients who died between 1994 and 1998 with asthma mentioned in part I of the death certificate. For each asthma death, a similar asthma admission (without death) was identified at the same hospital, with a similar admission date and a similar age.

Example: In a study of vascular dementia (Chan Carusone 2004), researchers selected 28 patients with vascular dementia who were enrolled in the Geriatric Clinic at Henderson Hospital in Hamilton, Ontario, between July 1999 and October 2001. They also selected controls from a list of all caregivers at that clinic, regardless of the diagnosis of their spouse or family member, as long as the caregiver did not have any signs of dementia or stroke. Caregivers were matched by age (within 5 years) and sex. The researchers tested both cases and controls for *Chlamydia*.

A case-control study is very efficient in studying rare diseases. With this design, you round up all of the limited number of cases of the disease and then find a comparable control group. By contrast, a cohort design has to round up far more exposures to ensure that a handful of them will develop the rare disease.

Case-control studies do not perform well when you are evaluating a diagnostic test. They are easy to set up, because you have a group of patients with the disease and you estimate the probability of a positive result for the diagnostic test in this group (sensitivity). You also have a control group and you estimate the probability of a negative result for the diagnostic test in this group (specificity). Unfortunately, the case-control design usually has a collection of very obviously diseased patients among the cases and very obviously healthy patients among the controls. This is an example of spectrum bias (Ransohoff 1978)—the lack of patients in the ambiguous middle of the spectrum. A study with spectrum bias will often overstate the sensitivity and specificity of a diagnostic test.

Example: A study of the rapid dipstick test for urinary tract infection (Lachs 1992), the sensitivity of the test was very good (92%) when restricted to a sample of patients with obvious signs of infection, but was poor (56%) when patients with more subtle manifestations of the disease were evaluated.

The case-control study is always retrospective because the outcome in a case-control study has already occurred. Retrospective studies usually have more problems with data quality because our memory is not always perfect. What is worse is that sometimes the ability to remember is sharply influenced by the outcome being studied. People who experience a tragic event like a miscarriage will have a strong desire to try to understand why this has happened and will search their past for risk factors that have been highly publicized in the press (Bryant 1989). They do not make things up, but the problem is that the people in the control group only seem to remember about half the things that have happened in their past. This selective under-reporting in the control group is known as recall bias and it can lead to some seriously faulty findings.

If you have 'leaky groups' in a case-control design, this can cause problems also. Do some of the disease outcomes get left out of the cases? It might be harder, for example, to identify the less serious examples of a disease. Patients with milder forms of Alzheimer's disease may not bother to seek out help. Only when the disease progresses enough to interfere with these patients' ability to live and function independently will you encounter such patients. Watch out also for situations where healthy people or people with the incorrect disease are accidentally classified as cases. You can avoid problems with leaky groups if there is some type of registry that allows the researchers to identify every possible case.

The other major problem with this type of study is that it is so hard to find a good control group. You want to find controls that are identical to the cases in all aspects except for the outcome itself. When there is a roster of all potentially eligible subjects (subjects who would be classified as cases if they developed the disease), then selection of a good control group is easy (Wacholder 1995). Most studies would not have such a roster. In this case, the controls are often patients admitted to the hospital for outcomes unrelated to the study. So if cases represent newly diagnosed lung cancer, then the controls might be patients admitted for a bone fracture. Other times, you might ask the case to bring a friend with them or to identify a relative.

Selection of controls in a case-control study is difficult enough, but you also have to worry about the selection of the cases. Do you select incident cases (e.g. all breast cancer patients newly diagnosed during a given time frame) or prevalent cases (e.g. all breast cancer patients who are alive during a given time frame)?

Selecting prevalent cases can lead to a very different answer than selecting incident cases. The probability of finding a case in a given time frame is related to mortality risk. Those patients who have a mild form of disease and survive for a relatively long time have a good chance of being around on the date that you go looking for them. Those patients who die quickly are unlikely to be around on the date that you go looking for them. A hypothetical example (Grimes 2002) involves a study of the relationship between snow shoveling and heart attacks. If such a study were done in a hospital setting, it would miss all the cases that died in their driveways. In general, selection of prevalent cases will lead to the selection of the milder and less rapidly fatal forms of the disease. A more detailed discussion of prevalence and incidence appears in Chapter 6.

Finally, the case-control design just does not sit well with your intuition. You are trying to find factors that cause an outcome, so you are sampling from the causes while a cohort design samples from the effects. Don't let this bother you too much, though. The mathematics that justify the case-control design were developed half a century ago (Cornfield 1951) and careful use of the case-control design has helped answer important clinical questions which could not have been answered by other research designs. Case-control designs, for example, established the use of aspirin as a cause of Reye's syndrome (Monto 1999). It is hard to imagine how a randomized trial for Reye's syndrome could have been done, because you would have to tell parents that you suspected, but were not quite sure, that giving an aspirin to a feverish child might lead to some pretty bad outcomes. So would you mind terribly if we recruited your son/daughter to participate in a trial where there is a 50% chance that they would get this possibly harmful substance?

1.4.3   The cross-sectional study

In contrast to the cohort and the case-control design, the cross-sectional study[3] selects on the basis of neither exposure nor outcome. With the cross-sectional design, you select a single group of patients and simultaneously assess both their exposure variables and their outcome variables.

Example: In a study of intimate partner violence (Malcoe 2004), 312 Native American women attending a tribally operated clinic filled out a survey form. The survey included a modified Conflict Tactics Scale to assess whether the women experienced verbal or psychological aggression, or physical or sexual assault. The survey also asked about educational attainment, employment status, receipt of food stamps, and other questions to help determine their socioeconomic status. Since both the outcome (intimate partner violence) and the exposure (socioeconomic status) were determined at the same time, this represents a cross-sectional survey.

Example: In a study of respiratory problems (Salo 2004), 5,051 seventh-grade students in Wuhan, China, completed a self-administered questionnaire. These students were classified according to six respiratory outcomes (wheezing with colds, wheezing without colds, bringing up phlegm with colds, bringing up phlegm without colds, coughing with colds, coughing without colds) and two exposure variables (coal burning for cooking and cleaning, and smoking in the home). Students were not randomly assigned to an exposure; so this is an observational study. Both the outcome variables and the exposure variables were assessed at a single point in time, so this represents a cross-sectional study.

Since there is no separation in time between assessment of exposure and assessment of outcome, you often cannot determine which came first. This loss of temporality makes it difficult to infer a cause-and-effect

---

[3] A lot of books on research will intentionally contrast cross-sectional and longitudinal designs. I do not mention longitudinal designs explicitly in this section because these do not fit into the hierarchy as I have described it. In general, a longitudinal design is usually a cohort design, with evaluation of the outcome at multiple time points. As such, it shares all the strengths and weaknesses of the cohort design. An additional strength of the longitudinal design, though, is that you can often gain considerable power for comparisons within a patient because you have removed between-patient variability from the equation. In this sense it is much like the crossover designs discussed in section 1.5.5.

relationship. A hypothetical example of patient height (Mann 2003) describes how a cross-sectional study might point up a negative association between height and age. Could this be because people shrink as they age, or perhaps successive generations of people are taller because of the improvements in nutrition, or perhaps taller people just die earlier? With a cross-sectional study, you cannot easily disentangle these alternate explanations.

Be cautious about leaky groups again. Will the selection process in a cross-sectional study correctly identify exposures and outcomes? In particular, are patients with more serious illnesses easier/harder to capture in the cross-sectional study than patients with milder forms of the illness?

Cross-sectional studies are fast, though, as you do not have to wait around to see what happens to the patients. These studies also allow you to easily explore relationships between multiple exposure variables and/or multiple outcome variables. But unlike the cohort design, which is useful for rare exposures, or the case-control design, which is useful for rare outcomes, the cross-sectional study is only effective if both the exposure and the outcome are relatively common events.

In general, the cross-sectional study is more useful as an exploratory tool, and can lead to the preparation of more definitive research studies with more rigorous designs.

1.4.4   The historical controls study

In a historical-control study, researchers will assign all of the research subjects to the new therapy. The outcomes of these subjects are compared to historical records representing the standard therapy.

Example: In a study of the rapid parathyroid hormone test (Johnson 2001), 49 patients undergoing parathyroidectomy received the rapid test. These patients were compared to 55 patients undergoing the same procedure before the rapid test was available. This is an observational study because the calendar, not the researchers, determined which test was applied. This particular observational study is a historical-control design because the control group represents patients tested before the availability of the rapid test.

The very nature of a historical-control study guarantees that there will be a major covariate imbalance between the two groups. Thus, you have to consider any factors that have changed over time that might be related to the outcome. To what extent might these factors affect the outcome differentially? For the most part, historical-control studies are considered one of the weakest forms of evidence. The one exception is when a disease has close to 100% mortality. In that situation, there is no need for a concurrent control group, since any therapy that is remotely effective can readily be detected. Even in this situation, you want to be sure that there is a biological basis for the treatment and that the disease group is homogeneous.

1.4.5 Nonrandomized studies: What to look for

For studies using a cohort design:

- Is the method for determining the exposure and control groups objective and accurate?
- Some covariate imbalances are inevitable, but are any of them serious?

For studies using a case-control design:

- Excluding the disease outcome itself, does the control group have similar features to the cases?
- Were some outcomes missed or were some healthy people accidentally included as cases?
- Is there a tendency for cases to have better recall of exposures than controls?

For studies using a cross-sectional design:

- Are patients with more serious disease harder to capture in this research design?
- Is there ambiguity about whether the exposure temporally precedes the disease?

For studies using a historical-control design:

- Did the authors provide a justification for this approach?
- In the time between the collection of the control group data and the treatment data, what other factors might have changed?

For all studies:

- How successful were the researchers in selecting a representative control group?
- Were there leaky groups? Were errors made in determining who had the exposure or who had the disease outcome?

1.5 Preventing covariate imbalance before it occurs

To ensure an apples-to-apples comparison, researchers will often use matching. Matching is the systematic selection, for every subject in the treatment/exposure group, of a control subject with similar characteristics. For example, in a study of fetal exposure to cocaine, you would select infants born to a mother who abused cocaine during pregnancy for your exposure group. For every such infant, you would select an infant unexposed to cocaine *in utero*, but also who had the same sex, race, and socioeconomic status for your control group.

Example: In a study of home versus hospital delivery (Ackerman-Liebrich 1996), 489 women who planned to deliver their babies at home were matched with women who planned to deliver at the hospital. Matching was based on age category (5 categories), parity category (3 categories), category of gynecological and obstetric history (24 categories or none), category of medical history (12 categories or none), social class (5 categories), and nationality. Because the matching criteria were so elaborate, they were only able to find a matched hospital delivery for about half of their home deliveries.

Matching will prevent covariate imbalance for those variables used in matching. It will also reduce covariate imbalance for any variables closely related to the matching variables. It will not, however, protect against all covariate imbalance, and covariates that are difficult to measure are especially problematic.

Matching often presents difficult logistical issues, because a matching control subject may not always be available. The logistics are especially difficult when there are several matching variables and when the pool of control subjects that you can draw from is not substantially larger than the pool of treatment/exposed subjects.

Matching is usually reserved for those variables that are known to be highly predictive of the outcome measure. In a cancer study, for example, matching is usually done on smoking. Many neonatology studies will match on gestational age.

1.5.1   Matching in a case-control design

When you are selecting patients on the basis of disease and looking back at what exposure might have caused the disease, selection of matching control patients (patients without disease) can sometimes be tricky. You need to find a control that is similar to the case, except for the disease of interest. There are several possibilities, but none of them work perfectly.

- You could recruit controls from undiseased members of the same family.
- You could ask each case to bring a friend with them. Their friend would be likely to be of similar age and socioeconomic status.
- You could find a control that lives in the same neighborhood as the case.
- You could find someone who visited the hospital at about the same time as the cases, but for a different reason.

Example: In a study of early onset myocardial infarction (Danesh 1999), 1,122 survivors of heart attacks in the age group of 30–49 were matched with people of the same age and gender who did not have heart attacks. These controls were recruited from a pool of subjects related to the cases. A second analysis used 510 survivors and their siblings, if the siblings were of the same sex and within five years of age of the survivor. All of the cases and the controls had blood tests to look for *Helicobacter pylori* infection, which was more commonly found in the cases than the controls.

Example: In a study of patients who leave a pediatric emergency department without being seen (Goldman 2005), patients who left were matched with the next two names on an alphabetical list of patients who visited on the same day and who had the same age (within one year), and the same sex. There was a large pool of controls to draw from, since patients who left comprised only 289 of the 11,087 total visitors.

1.5.2   Matching in a randomized design

In some randomized studies, matching will be used as well. Partly, this is a recognition that randomization will not totally remove covariate imbalance; just as a flip of 100 coins will not always result in exactly 50 heads and 50 tails. More importantly, however, matching in a randomized study will provide extra precision. Matching creates pairs of subjects who will have greater homogeneity and therefore less variability.

Example: In a study of a Mental Health First Aid course (Jorm 2004), sixteen local government areas in rural Australia were matched into pairs based on size, geography, and socioeconomic level. In each pair, one area was assigned to receive immediate training while the other was assigned to a waiting list.

1.5.3   Matching can sometimes backfire

Matching often presents difficult logistical issues, because a matching control subject may not always be available. The logistics are especially difficult when there are several matching variables and when the pool of control subjects that you can draw from is not substantially larger than the pool of treatment/exposed subjects.

In the tinnitus study mentioned above, although there were 1,121 patients, 143 of them did not have a close match in the data and were excluded from the matched analysis. There was also some attrition in the study, which caused a greater loss in the matched analysis. If one of the patients in a pair dropped out, the other patient's data could not be used in the matched analysis. So the analysis of improvement after 4 weeks included only 414 pairs and the analysis after 14 weeks included only 354 pairs. Although the loss in sample size was probably offset by the added precision from the matching, the authors do acknowledge that this was probably 'an unnecessary and disadvantageous complication'.

Contrast this, though, with the study of patients who left the ER. These patients represented less than 3% (289/11,087) of the total pool of subjects and this made it easy to find not just one, but two matching control patients.

In a case-control design, matching can sometimes remove the very effect you are trying to study. You should avoid matching when the matching variable is caused by the exposure or is a similar measure of exposure. This produces overmatching and ends up reducing the effect of the exposure. In a study examining radiation exposure and the risk of leukemia at a nuclear reprocessing plant (Marsh 2002), there were 37 workers diagnosed with leukemia (cases) and they were each matched to four control workers. Each of the four control workers had to work at the same site, be the same gender, have the same job code, be born within two years of the case, and had to be hired within two years of the hire date of the case.

Unfortunately, there was a strong trend between hire dates and exposures. Exposures were highest early in the plant's history and declined over time. So both hire date and exposure were measuring the same thing. When the data were matched on hire dates, it artefactually controlled the exposures and pretty much ensured that the average radiation exposure would be the same among both the cases and the controls. This led to an estimate of radiation exposure that was actually slightly negative and not statistically significant. When the data were rematched using all the variables except for hire date, the effect of radiation dose was large and positive and came close to approaching statistical significance.

1.5.4   Stratification

Stratification is a method similar to matching that tries to achieve covariate balance across broad groups or strata. The selection of subjects in both the treatment group and the control group are constrained to have identical proportions in each strata. This guarantees covariate balance for the strata itself and any other factors closely related to the strata.

Example: In a study of medical records (Fine 2003), 54 records were selected from each of ten cardiac surgery centers and were examined for accuracy and completeness. To ensure a good balance, the 54 records at each site were allocated evenly to six different predefined risk strata (nine in each strata).

Another use of stratification is to ensure that the sample has numbers in each strata that are proportional to numbers in the strata for the entire population of interest. This helps ensure that the sample is generalizable to the entire population.

Example: In a study of retention of doctors in rural Australia (Humphreys 2002), a random sample of 1,400 doctors was sent a questionnaire. The doctors were selected in strata defined by the size of the town where they lived.

This kept the proportion in each strata equivalent to those proportions in the entire population of Australian doctors.

The strata are usually broadly drawn. If there were a small number of possible patients within each strata, then the logistics become too difficult. So, for example, stratification by age will usually involve large intervals such as 21–30 years, 31–40 years, etc.

You cannot stratify on factors that you cannot measure or on information that is not immediately available at the start of the study. And like matching, stratification only works when you have a large pool of subjects to draw from.

Stratification can add precision to a randomized study. A separate randomization list would be drawn up for each strata. This would ensure that the strata would have perfect balance between the treatment group and the control group.

1.5.5   The crossover design

The crossover design represents a special type of matching. In a crossover design, a subject is randomly assigned to a specific treatment order. Some subjects will receive the standard therapy first, followed by the new therapy (AB). Others will receive the new therapy first, followed by the standard therapy (BA). Since the same subject receives both treatments, there is no possibility of covariate imbalance.

Example: In a study of electronic records (Brown 2003), ten physicians were asked to code patient records with two separate systems: Clinical Terms Version 3 and with the Read Codes 5 Byte Set. Half of the physicians were randomly assigned to code using Clinical Terms Version 3 first and then later with the Read Codes 5 Byte Set. The other half coded using Read Codes 5 Byte Set first.

When therapies are applied in sequence, timing effects are of great concern. Are the therapies set far apart enough so that the effect of one therapy is unlikely to carry over into the other therapy? For example, if the two therapies represent different drugs, did the researchers allow enough time so that one drug was fully eliminated from the body before they administered the second drug?

The washout period can sometimes cause ethical concerns. If you are treating patients for depression, an extensive amount of time during the washout would leave the patient without any effective treatment and increase the chances of something bad happening, like the patient committing suicide.

The possibility of learning effects are also potential problems in a crossover design. You cannot use a crossover design, for example, to test alternative training approaches. Imagine the instructions for this study (*now forget everything we just told you; we are going to teach it a different way*).

I guess that would work for the classes I teach; the only thing my students remember are the jokes.

Also, watch out for the possibility that a subject may get tired or bored. This could lead to the second treatment assigned being worse than the first. Or, if the outcome involves skill, maybe 'practice makes perfect' leading to the second treatment assigned being better than the first.

If there are timing effects, randomization is critical. Even with randomization, though, timing effects are a problem because they increase uncertainty by adding an extra source of variation.

Special problems arise when each subject always receives one therapy first and it is always followed by the other therapy. Many factors, other than the change in therapy, can cause a shift in the health of patients over time. If you cannot randomize the order of treatments, you have all the problems of a historical-control study.

1.5.6 Things to look for in a study with matching or stratification

When a study uses matching, look for the following features.
For a study using matching (stratification):

- Did the researchers match (stratify) on the most important covariates?
- Were the matching (stratification) variables measured accurately?
- Were any important variables not considered in the matching (stratification)?

For studies using a crossover design:

- Was the order of treatments randomized?
- Were there any carry-over effects?
- Were there any fatigue effects?

1.6   Statistical adjustments

Statistical adjustments represent one way of correcting for covariate imbalance. While matching and stratification, try to prevent covariate imbalance before it occurs, statistical adjustment corrects for the imbalance after the fact.

The best example I can find for covariate adjustment is a nonmedical example. You might still enjoy this example, though, if you have ever tried to buy a house. The data comes from the Data and Story Library[4] and shows

---

[4] The Data and Story Library is available at: www.lib.stat.cmu.edu/DASL/DataArchive.html. This particular data-set is available at: www.lib.stat.cmu.edu/DASL/Stories/ homeprice.html. There is a lot more going on with this data-set than I have discussed here, and if you are the ambitious sort, you should download this data-set and try a few additional data analyses yourself.

the housing prices of 117 homes in Albuquerque, New Mexico in 1993. The data-set also includes variables that might influence the sales price of the home such as the size in square feet, the age in years, and whether the house was custom-built (see Figure 1.1).

When you look at the average sales price for regular homes and custom built homes, you see a large discrepancy. Regular homes sell, on average for $95,000, but custom-built homes sell for $145,000 on average, a $50,000 discrepancy.

But when you draw a graph that shows both the size of the house and the price (see graph), you notice that custom-built houses (denoted by C on the graph) are not all that much different from the regular houses (denoted by R). The margins of the graph explain exactly what is happening. On the right-hand side, you see a box plot for the prices of regular and custom homes. The plus signs inside each box plot represent the mean prices. When you look at this dimension alone, the prices seem quite different. At the bottom of the graph are box plots for the size of the homes. Uh-oh! It looks like the custom-built homes are quite a bit bigger than the regular homes (2,100 versus 1,500 square feet). This is hardly surprising. People who have the money for custom-builts also have the money for a roomier and more spacious house.

So now you have to wonder—are custom-builts more expensive because they are custom-builts or just because they are bigger? This is the sort of confusion you always have to deal with when you encounter covariate imbalance. The solution is to adjust for the differences in house sizes.

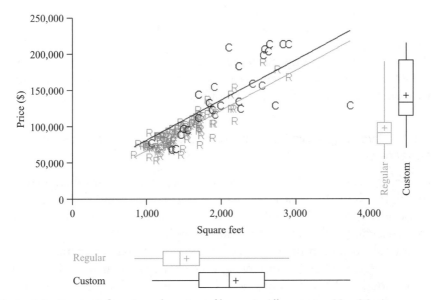

Figure 1.1   Factors influencing sales prices of homes in Albuquerque, New Mexico.

There is a fairly strong and predictable relationship between size and price. For every extra square foot of space, the average sales price increases by $55. Multiply this by 600 square feet, the discrepancy in sizes between the average custom-built and the average regular home. It turns out that of the $50,000 gap that you observed, $33,000 can be explained by the difference in average sizes. The remaining $17,000 is probably real. So a covariate adjustment would reduce the estimated difference in prices by about 2/3.

The trend lines in the plot above shows the relationship between size and price and the gap between the lines represents the difference in price adjusting for size. So, for example, a house with 2,000 square feet would sell for an estimated $137,000 if it were custom-built and around $120,000 if it were not.

Example: A study of males residents of Caerphilly, South Wales (Smith 1997) examined the relationship between frequency of orgasm and ten-year mortality. They divided the men into low, medium, and high frequency of orgasm. Low frequency meant less than monthly and high frequency meant twice a week or more often. This is a study which would have been impossible to randomize—the men (and presumably their wives) determined their group membership. As you might expect, there were demographic differences in the three groups. Age was significantly associated with frequency of orgasm. Men in the low, medium, and high frequency groups were 54, 52, and 50 years old, on average. The job categories also differed, with the proportion of nonmanual labor being 29%, 42%, and 42% among the three groups. For other variables (height, body mass index, systolic blood pressure, cholesterol, existing coronary heart disease, and smoking status), the differences were smaller and less important. The adjustments used a combination of regression approaches and weighting. After adjustment, there was a strong trend in mortality, with men in the low frequency group having an adjusted mortality rate that was twice as big as the high frequency group. Both the article itself, and a subsequent letter to the editor (Batty 1998) mentioned, however, that additional unmeasured variables could have influenced the outcome.

1.6.1   Avoiding covariate imbalance by looking at a special subgroup

If there is covariate imbalance in the entire sample, perhaps there may be a subgroup where the covariate is balanced. If you can find such a subgroup and it produces results similar to the entire sample, you can have greater confidence in the findings of the entire sample.

Example: In a study of the effect of men's age on time to pregnancy (Hassan 2003), older men tended to have a longer time to pregnancy. These older men, though, also have older wives, on average. This creates an unfair comparison, since the wife's age would probably also influence time to pregnancy. To produce a fairer comparison, they conducted a separate analysis looking at men of all ages who married young wives.

Of course, it is not always possible to find a subgroup without covariate imbalance. And when you do find such a subgroup, the smaller sample size may lead to an unacceptable loss of precision. Furthermore, the subgroup may be somewhat unusual, making it difficult for you to generalize the findings.

1.6.2   Reweighting to restore balance

Another way to restore balance in a study is the use of weights. Suppose the treatment group includes 25 males and 75 females, but in population we know that there should be a 50/50 split by gender. We could reweight the data, so that each male has a weighting factor of 2.0 and each female has a weighting factor of 0.67. This artificially inflates the number of males to 50 and deflates the number of females to 50. The control group might have 40 males and 60 females. For this group, we would use weights of 1.25 and 0.83.

A recent article on educational testing (Wainer 2004) shows how a simple reweighting of the data can lead to a fairer comparison between two groups. These researchers show data on a state by state basis for the National Assessment of Educational Progress (NAEP). Two states, Nebraska and New Jersey, show interesting results. The average score for Nebraska is 277 and only 271 for New Jersey. But, interestingly enough, New Jersey outperforms Nebraska among whites (283 vs. 281), blacks (242 vs. 236) and other nonwhite (260 vs. 259).

This odd finding occurs because New Jersey has much different demographics than Nebraska. In New Jersey 66% of the population is white, 15% black, and 19% other nonwhite. In Nebraska, 87% of the population is white, 5% black, and 8% other nonwhite. It is this differing demographic mix that causes the paradox.

The average score for each state is a weighted average. For Nebraska, the calculation is

$$281*0.87 + 236*0.05 + 259*0.08 = 277$$

and for New Jersey, the calculation is

$$283*0.66 + 242*0.15 + 260*0.19 = 272.$$

Nebraska benefits because a higher weight (0.87) is placed on the race that scored highest in both states. What would happen to Nebraska's and New Jersey's scores if the demographic mix was changed to the overall percentages in the United States. (69% white, 16% black, and 15% other nonwhite)?

Here are the reweighted calculations for Nebraska:

$$281*0.69 + 236*0.16 + 259*0.15 = 271$$

and New Jersey:

$$283*0.69 + 242*0.16 + 260*0.15 = 273.$$

My numbers do not match perfectly with the original article because of rounding error, but the overall conclusions remain the same. Nebraska does have a higher mean than New Jersey but when you adjust this mean for the racial demographics, New Jersey actually does better.

Reweighting to a common demographic risk is often used to make adjustments between two groups that have sharply differing mixes of age, gender, and/or racial characteristics.

The statistical analysis gets a bit tricky with weights, but nothing that a professional statistician cannot handle. Weights can also improve the generalizability of a study. If the overall sample has a skewed demographic, weights can help bring it back in line with the population of interest.

1.6.3 Unmeasured covariates

You can only adjust for those things that you can measure. Unfortunately, there are many things such as a patient's psychological state, presence of co-morbid conditions, and initial severity of the disease that are so difficult to assess that they are often just not measured.

Example: A study of asthma and chronic obstructive pulmonary disease in several different data sources (Hansell 2003), showed inconsistent results for asthma across the data sources. The authors speculate that smoking and social class might influence these results, but these variables were not available in most of the data-sets used in this study.

Example: A study of hip fractures (Ray 2002), noted that three previous case-control studies using large databases had suggested that statins were associated with a lower risk of hip fractures among elderly patients. The authors speculated that there may be a 'healthy drug user effect' that would bias these findings. By a healthy drug effect, the authors meant that patients who use preventive measures and comply with them faithfully are likely to be less seriously ill at baseline than patients who do not take preventive measures or are poor compliers. Some of this may be that these patients just have better general self-care habits. In addition, doctors might be more likely to prescribe statins to heavier patients and the extra padding in these patients provides some protection against hip fracture. Measuring self-care habits would be impossible to do in most research settings, but especially in a retrospective study like a case-control design. Patient weights are easier to obtain, but unfortunately, these data were not available in two of the three case-control studies. The authors conducted a cohort study, which had some of the same problems as the case-control studies because it, too, was retrospective and had no data on patient weights. Nevertheless, the fact that patients using statins and patients using other lipid lowering drugs, both had comparable levels of reduced hip fractures compared to nonusers, which indicated that it might be an overall effect of healthy lifestyles of patients that use any preventive medicine rather than the effect of the statins themselves that reduced the risk of hip fractures.

1.6.4 Imperfectly measured covariates

Some covariates can be measured, but only crudely. If the covariate itself is difficult to measure accurately, then any attempts to make statistical adjustments will only be partially successful. Your measurement may only capture half of the information in the covariate. The half of the covariate that is unaccounted for will remain behind, leading to an unfair comparison. This is sometimes called residual confounding.

Example: In a study of factors influencing Down's syndrome (Chen 1999), smoking had a surprisingly protective effect. This could be explained by the age of the mother. Older mothers smoke less and are also at greater risk for birth of a Down's syndrome child. The unadjusted odds ratio for this effect was 0.80 and was borderline statistically significant (95% CI, 0.65–0.98). A crude adjustment for age used the categories <35 years and >35 years. With this adjustment, the odds ratio was still small (0.87) and borderline (95% CI, 0.71–1.07). But when the exact year of age was used to adjust, and race and parity were also included in the adjustment, there was no association (odds ratio=1.00, 95% CI, 0.82–1.24). This shows that an imperfect adjustment can produce an incorrect conclusion.

Example: In a study of adverse birth outcomes (Elliott 2001), residents who lived within two kilometers of a landfill site were compared to more distant individuals. The authors acknowledged that these landfills were typically located in areas that were already poverty stricken. So perhaps factors associated with poverty, such as poorer nutrition, might influence the risk of adverse birth outcomes rather than the landfill itself. They tried to account for poverty using the Carstairs index, a measure of deprivation. The authors admit that this is a rather crude adjustment, and perhaps some additional degree of poverty was left unaccounted for. An accompanying editorial (McNamee 2001) pointed out that even a 10% disparity in a risk factor that doubles the chances of an adverse birth outcome could lead to changes that dwarf the effects seen in this particular study.

Self-report measures are often measured imperfectly, and are especially troublesome if they require the patient to recall events from the distant past.

Smoking is an important covariate for many studies and it would be better to ask about the amount of smoking for current smokers. For smokers who have quit recently, you might also like to know how recently they quit. For both groups it might also help know when they started. But often, the only question asked is a yes/no question like 'Do you smoke cigarettes?'

Some covariates like blood cholesterol levels are inherently variable. In an ideal world, these covariates would be measured at a second time and the two measures could be averaged to reduce some of the uncertainty. But this is not always possible or practical.

1.6.5   Adjusting for variables in the causal pathway

Although adjusting for covariate imbalance is usually a good thing, you can sometimes take it too far. If your treatment influences an intermediate variable and that variable influences the outcome, then the intermediate variable is said to be in the causal pathway.

For example, I was coauthor on a research study (Kliethermes 1999) that was trying to improve rate of breastfeeding in a group of preterm infants. The intervention was to feed these infants, when the mother was not around, through their nasogastric tube. This sounds like an icky thing, but remember that the population is preterm infants, who probably have to have an nasogastric tube anyway. So it would not be too weird to use this tube for feeding. It might mean that the nasogastric tube would have to stay in a bit longer, but if this lead to a greater proportion of mothers breastfeeding at three and six months, that would be a worthwhile tradeoff.

In the control group, infants would be fed from a bottle when the mother was not around. For both groups, of course, breastfeeding would be encouraged whenever the mother was with the baby. Keep in mind that these are preterm babies, so some of them may stay in the hospital for weeks. Since the mothers left the hospital much sooner than their babies, what to do while the mother was not around was very critical.

It turns out that the intervention was very successful. Infants randomized to the nasogastric tube feeding group had higher rates of breastfeeding at discharge, three days post discharge, as well as at three and six months. One possible explanation for this success is that infants who receive too many bottles early in life may have trouble latching onto the mother's nipple.

When the researchers collected the data, they included a variable which measured the number of bottles of formula received during the hospital stay. This variable was zero for most of the infants in the nasogastric tube feeding group, although a handful of infants in this group did incorrectly get a few bottles of formula.

Just on a whim, I decided to adjust for the number of bottles received. I was shocked to find out that the effect of the treatment disappeared when I adjusted for the number of bottles. At first, I panicked, but then I realized that this adjustment, if anything, proved the effectiveness of the intervention. The number of bottles received was directly influenced by the intervention, and the fact that this intermediate variable was more strongly associated with breastfeeding rates than the intervention itself should not come as a surprise.

We did not publish the results of this particular analysis, partly for space limitations and partly because it was difficult to explain properly. But I took it as a lesson to think carefully about covariate adjustment, and not to just toss a variable into the fray.

1.6.6   Adjustments: What to look for

If a study uses covariate adjustments, look for the following things:

- Did the study adjust on variables that are truly important to the outcome?
- Were the variables used in adjustment measured accurately?
- Were there unmeasured covariates that could have influenced the outcome?

1.7   Counterpoint: Randomized trials are overrated

Can matching and/or statistical adjustments in an observational study provide a comparison as fair and as persuasive as a randomized study? This is an unfair question, because sometimes a randomized study is just not possible. Also, there are so many different types of observational studies that it would be difficult to come up with a good general answer. Still, some people have tried to answer this question.

An empirical study of observational and randomized studies of the same topic (Concato 2000) found that there was a high level of consistency between the two. This contradicted the previously held belief that observational studies tended to overstate the effectiveness of a new treatment. The debate about this finding continues to rage, but perhaps the quality of the design and the sophistication of the adjustments used in observational studies places them on a level comparable to randomized studies. A study on thrombolytic treatment in patients with acute myocardial infarction (Koch 1997) showed that a large nonrandomized registry provided data that were comparable to that collected in randomized studies.

Randomized studies have some additional weaknesses. The very process of randomization will create an artificial environment that does not represent how medicine is normally practiced (Sackett 1997). When you go to your doctor for assistance with birth control, you do not expect him/her to randomly assign you to a particular method. And if your doctor said you had a 50% chance of getting a placebo contraceptive, you would probably switch doctors. Because an observational study does not have to cope with the intrusion of the randomization process, it can often study medicine in an environment much closer to reality. Furthermore, the use of a placebo in a randomized trial creates an artificial situation where patients are more likely to drop out and less likely to report side effects (Rochon 1999).

Another problem with randomized designs is the limit to their size and scope. The logistics of randomization make it more expensive than a comparable observational study. Thus effects that require a very large sample size to detect (such as rare side effects) or effects that take a long time to manifest themselves (such as the progression of many types of cancer) cannot be examined in a randomized experiment. An observational approach, like post-marketing surveillance, is more likely to be successful in these situations.

All other things being equal, a randomized study provides a higher standard of evidence than an observational study, but rarely are all other things equal.

1.8   Summary—Apples or oranges?

Make sure that your control group represents a fair comparison.

Was randomization used? Randomization ensures balance on average across both measured and unmeasured covariates.

If randomization was not possible, to what extent did covariate imbalance occur? We there errors in assessing exposure status and/or in determining the outcome?

If matching or statistical adjustments were used, did these incorporate covariates that were truly important to the outcome? Were these covariates measured accurately?

1.9   On your own

1. Review the following abstracts, all from studies where randomization was not done. Speculate on the reason that randomization was not performed.

Body fatness during childhood and adolescence and incidence of breast cancer in premenopausal women: a prospective cohort study. Baer, H.J., Colditz, G.A., Rosner, B., Michels, K.B., Rich-Edwards, J.W., Hunter, D.J., and Willett, W.C. *Breast Cancer Research* 2005, 7:R314–R325 doi:10.1186/bcr998. **Introduction:** Body mass index (BMI) during adulthood is inversely related to the incidence of premenopausal breast cancer, but the role of body fatness earlier in life is less clear. We examined prospectively the relation between body fatness during childhood and adolescence and the incidence of breast cancer in premenopausal women. **Methods:** Participants were 109,267 premenopausal women in the Nurses' Health Study II who recalled their body fatness at ages 5, 10 and 20 years using a validated 9-level figure drawing. Over 12 years of follow-up, 1,318 incident cases of breast cancer were identified. Cox proportional hazards regression was used to compute relative risks (RRs) and 95% confidence intervals (CIs) for body fatness at each age and for average childhood (ages 5–10 years) and adolescent (ages 10–20 years) fatness. **Results:** Body fatness at each age was inversely associated with premenopausal breast cancer incidence; the multivariate RRs were 0.48 (95% CI, 0.35–0.55) and 0.57 (95% CI, 0.39–0.83) for the most overweight compared with the most lean in childhood and adolescence, respectively (p for trend < 0.0001). The association for childhood body fatness was only slightly attenuated after adjustment for later BMI, with a multivariate RR of 0.52 (95% CI, 0.38–0.71) for the most overweight compared with the most lean (p for trend = 0.001). Adjustment for menstrual cycle characteristics had little impact on the association. **Conclusion:** Greater body fatness during childhood and adolescence is associated with reduced incidence of premenopausal breast cancer, independent of adult BMI and menstrual cycle characteristics.

This is an open source publication. The full free text is available at: www.breast-cancer-research.com/content/7/3/R314.

Impact of a nurses' protocol-directed weaning procedure on outcomes in patients undergoing mechanical ventilation for longer than 48 hours: a prospective cohort study with a matched historical control group. Tonnelier, J.-M., Prat, G., Le Gal, G., Gut-Gobert, C., Renault, A., Boles, J.-M., and L'Her, E. *Critical Care* 2005, 9:R83–R89 doi:10.1186/cc3030. **Introduction:** The aim of the study was to determine whether the use of a nurses' protocol-directed weaning procedure, based on the French intensive care society (SRLF) consensus recommendations, was associated with reductions in the duration of mechanical ventilation and intensive care unit (ICU) length of stay in patients requiring more than 48 hours of mechanical ventilation. **Methods:** This prospective study was conducted in a university hospital ICU from January 2002 through to February 2003. A total of 104 patients who had been ventilated for more than 48 hours and were weaned from mechanical ventilation using a nurses' protocol-directed procedure (cases) were compared with a 1:1 matched historical control group who underwent conventional physician-directed weaning (between 1999 and 2001). Duration of ventilation and length of ICU stay, rate of unsuccessful extubation and rate of ventilator-associated pneumonia were compared between cases and controls. **Results:** The duration of mechanical ventilation (16.6 ± 13 days versus 22.5 ± 21 days; p = 0.02) and ICU length of stay (21.6 ± 14.3 days versus 27.6 ± 21.7 days; p = 0.02) were lower among patients who underwent the nurses' protocol-directed weaning than among control individuals. Ventilator-associated pneumonia, ventilator discontinuation failure rates and ICU mortality were similar between the two groups. **Discussion:** Application of the nurses' protocol-directed weaning procedure described here is safe and promotes significant outcome benefits in patients who require more than 48 hours of mechanical ventilation.

This is an open source publication. The full free text is available at: www.ccforum.com/content/9/2/R83.

Extravascular lung-water in patients with severe sepsis: a prospective cohort study. Martin, G.S., Eaton, S., Mealer, M., and Moss, M. *Critical Care* 2005, 9:R74–R82 doi:10.1186/cc3025. **Introduction:** Few investigations have prospectively examined extravascular lung water (EVLW) in patients with severe sepsis. We sought to determine whether EVLW may contribute to lung injury in these patients by quantifying the relationship of EVLW to parameters of lung injury, to determine the effects of chronic alcohol abuse on EVLW, and to determine whether EVLW may be a useful tool in the diagnosis of acute respiratory distress syndrome (ARDS). **Methods:** The present prospective cohort study was conducted in consecutive patients with severe sepsis from a medical intensive care unit in an urban university teaching hospital. In each patient, transpulmonary thermodilution was used to measure cardiovascular hemodynamics and EVLW for 7 days via an arterial catheter placed within 72 hours of meeting criteria for severe sepsis. **Results:** A total of 29 patients were studied. Twenty-five of the 29 patients (86%) were mechanically ventilated, 15 of the 29 patients (52%) developed ARDS, and overall 28-day mortality was 41%. Eight out of 14 patients (57%) with non-ARDS severe sepsis had high EVLW with significantly greater hypoxemia than did those patients with low EVLW (mean arterial oxygen tension/fractional inspired oxygen ratio 230.7 $\pm$ 36.1 mmHg versus 341.2$\pm$92.8 mmHg; $p<0.001$). Four out of 15 patients with severe sepsis with ARDS maintained a low EVLW and had better 28-day survival than did ARDS patients with high EVLW (100% versus 36%; $p = 0.03$). ARDS patients with a history of chronic alcohol abuse had greater EVLW than did nonalcoholic patients (19.9 ml/kg versus 8.7 ml/kg; $p<0.0001$). The arterial oxygen tension/fractional inspired oxygen ratio, lung injury score, and chest radiograph scores correlated with EVLW (r^2= 0.27, r^2=0.18, and r^2=0.28, respectively; all $p<0.0001$). **Conclusions:** More than half of the patients with severe sepsis but without ARDS had increased EVLW, possibly representing subclinical lung injury. Chronic alcohol abuse was associated with increased EVLW, whereas lower EVLW was associated with survival. EVLW correlated moderately with the severity of lung injury but did not account for all respiratory derangements. EVLW may improve both risk stratification and management of patients with severe sepsis.

This is an open source publication. The full free text is available at: www.ccforum.com/content/9/2/R74.

Breast implants following mastectomy in women with early-stage breast cancer: prevalence and impact on survival. Le, G.M., O'Malley, C.D.,

Glaser, S.L., Lynch, C.F., Stanford, J.L., Keegan, T.H.M., and West, D.W. *Breast Cancer Research* 2005, 7:R184–R193 doi:10.1186/bcr974. **Background:** Few studies have examined the effect of breast implants after mastectomy on long-term survival in breast cancer patients, despite growing public health concern over potential long-term adverse health effects. **Methods:** We analyzed data from the Surveillance, Epidemiology and End Results Breast Implant Surveillance Study conducted in San Francisco–Oakland, in Seattle–Puget Sound, and in Iowa. This population-based, retrospective cohort included women younger than 65 years when diagnosed with early or unstaged first primary breast cancer between 1983 and 1989, treated with mastectomy. The women were followed for a median of 12.4 years ($n = 4,968$). Breast implant usage was validated by medical record review. Cox proportional hazards models were used to estimate hazard rate ratios for survival time until death due to breast cancer or other causes for women with and without breast implants, adjusted for relevant patient and tumor characteristics. **Results:** Twenty percent of cases received postmastectomy breast implants, with silicone gel-filled implants comprising the most common type. Patients with implants were younger and more likely to have *in situ* disease than patients not receiving implants. Risks of breast cancer mortality (hazard ratio, 0.54; 95% CI, 0.43–0.67) and nonbreast cancer mortality (hazard ratio, 0.59; 95% CI, 0.41–0.85) were lower in patients with implants than in those patients without implants, following adjustment for age and year of diagnosis, race/ethnicity, stage, tumor grade, histology, and radiation therapy. Implant type did not appear to influence long-term survival. **Conclusions:** In a large, population-representative sample, breast implants following mastectomy do not appear to confer any survival disadvantage following early-stage breast cancer in women younger than 65 years old.

This is an open source publication. The full free text is available at: www.breast-cancer-research.com/content/7/2/R184.

Pregnancy weight gain and breast cancer risk. Kinnunen, T.I., Luoto, R., Gissler, M., Hemminki E., and Hilakivi-Clarke, L. *BMC Women's Health* 2004, 4:7 doi:10.1186/1472-6874-4-7. **Background:** Elevated pregnancy estrogen levels are associated with increased risk of developing breast cancer in mothers. We studied whether pregnancy weight gain that has been linked to high circulating estrogen levels, affects a mother's breast cancer risk. **Methods:** Our cohort consisted of women who were pregnant between 1954 and 1963 in Helsinki, Finland, of whom 2,089 were eligible for the study. Pregnancy data were collected from patient records of maternity centers. As many as 123 subsequent breast cancer cases were identified through a record linkage to the Finnish Cancer Registry, and the mean age at diagnosis was 56 years (range 35–74). A sample of 979 women (123 cases, 856 controls) from the cohort was linked to the Hospital Inpatient

Registry to obtain information on the women's stay in hospitals. **Results:** Mothers in the upper tertile of pregnancy weight gain (>15 kg) had a 1.62-fold (95% CI, 1.03–2.53) higher breast cancer risk than mothers who gained the recommended amount (the middle tertile, mean: 12.9 kg, range 11–15 kg), after adjusting for mother's age at menarche, age at first birth, age at index pregnancy, parity at the index birth, and body mass index (BMI) before the index pregnancy. In a separate nested case-control study ($n = 65$ cases and 431 controls), adjustment for BMI at the time of breast cancer diagnosis did not modify the findings. **Conclusions:** Our study suggests that high pregnancy weight gain increases later breast cancer risk, independently from body weight at the time of diagnosis.

This is an open source publication. The full free text is available at: www.biomedcentral.com/1472-6874/4/7.

Racial variations in processes of care for patients with community-acquired pneumonia. Mortensen, E.M., Cornell, J., and Whittle, J. *BMC Health Services Research* 2004, 4:20 doi:10.1186/1472-6963-4-20. **Background:** Patients hospitalized with community acquired pneumonia (CAP) have a substantial risk of death, but there is evidence that adherence to certain processes of care, including antibiotic administration within 8 hours, can decrease this risk. Although national mortality data show blacks have a substantially increased odds of death due to pneumonia as compared to whites previous studies of short-term mortality have found decreased mortality for blacks. Therefore we examined pneumonia-related processes of care and short-term mortality in a population of patients hospitalized with CAP. **Methods:** We reviewed the records of all identified Medicare beneficiaries hospitalized for pneumonia between October 1, 1998 and September 30, 1999 at one of 101 Pennsylvania hospitals, and randomly selected 60 patients at each hospital for inclusion. We reviewed the medical records to gather process measures of quality, pneumonia severity and demographics. We used Medicare administrative data to identify 30-day mortality. Because only a small proportion of the study population was black, we included all 240 black patients and randomly selected 720 white patients matched on age and gender. We performed a resampling of the white patients 10 times. **Results:** Males were 43% of the cohort, and the median age was 76 years. After controlling for potential confounders, blacks were less likely to receive antibiotics within 8 hours (odds ratio with 95% CI, 0.6, 0.4–0.97), but were as likely as whites to have blood cultures obtained before receiving antibiotics (0.7, 0.3–1.5), to have oxygenation assessed within 24 hours of presentation (1.6, 0.9–3.0), and to receive guideline concordant antibiotics (OR 0.9, 0.6–1.7). Black patients had a trend towards decreased 30-day mortality (0.4, 0.2 to 1.0). **Conclusion:** Although blacks were less likely to receive optimal care, our findings are consistent with other studies that suggest better risk-adjusted survival among blacks than among whites. Further study is needed to determine why this is the case.

This is an open source publication. The full free text is available at www.biomedcentral.com/1472-6963/4/20.

For each of the abstracts shown above, classify the study as a cohort study, case-control study, cross-sectional study, or historical-control study.

2 Who Was Left Out? Exclusions, Refusals, and Dropouts

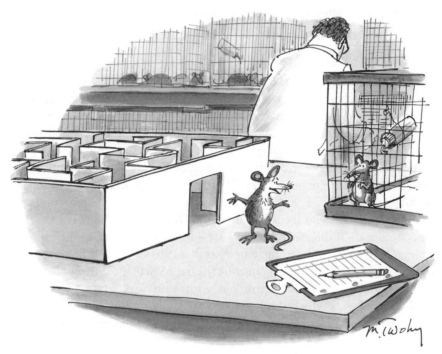

"I don't usually volunteer for experiments, but I'm kind of a puzzle freak."

2.1 Introduction

Research studies often have a narrow focus, but sometimes it can be too narrow. When too many patients are left out, those who remain may not be representative of the types of patients you will encounter.

2.1.1 Case study: Nicotine patches

In a study of teenage smokers (Smith 1996), researchers recruited volunteers each from five public high schools in Rochester, Minnesota, for participation in a smoking cessation program involving behavioral counseling, group therapy, and nicotine patches. Researchers measured the number of cigarettes smoked, side effects, and blood levels of nicotine.

The purpose of the research was to evaluate 'the safety, tolerance, and efficacy of 22 mg/d nicotine patch therapy in smokers younger than 18 years who were trying to stop smoking.' The authors also listed a secondary goal, 'to compare blood cotinine levels, nicotine withdrawal scores, and adverse experiences with those of adults obtained in previous patch studies.' Cotinine is a metabolite of nicotine and provides a useful objective measure of cigarette smoking. The study allowed the authors to examine whether nicotine toxicity was an issue.

This study did not include major segments of the teenage smoking population. It included only white subjects because there were too few minority students in Rochester. Subjects had to get parental permission, excluding smokers who wished to keep their habit secret from their parents. Subjects were also volunteers, and thus could be considered more motivated to quit than the typical teenage smoker.

The study also had a serious dropout rate. Of the presumably thousands of teenage smokers in Rochester only 71 volunteers responded to the initial call for subjects. Of the 71, 55% met inclusion criteria. Of the remaining 39, 44% declined to attend the initial meeting. Of the remaining 22, 14% were noncompliant. Of the remaining 18, 39% failed to respond to the one-year survey. Only 11 completed the entire study (50% of those who started the study; 28% of those meeting inclusion criteria; 15% of the initial volunteers).

This study had a serious problem with who was left out. The large number of subjects who did not get into the study or who did not complete the study makes it hard to generalize the findings of this research.

2.1.2   Who was left out? What to look for

When you are trying to figure out who was left out and what impact this has, ask the following questions:

Who was excluded at the start of the study? In a desire to create a nice clean homogeneous research study, researchers may apply rigid and unrealistic entry criteria. The patients excluded can often have a different prognosis than those who make it into the study. This exclusion can make it difficult to extrapolate to the types of patients that you normally see.

Who refused to join the study? Almost all research involves the informed consent of volunteers. Many potential patients can and do refuse to participate in research studies. This can dramatically affect the results of the research.

Who dropped out during the study? Not everyone who starts out in a research study will finish it. Volunteers always have the option of withdrawing their consent to participate at any time and some patients will miss their follow-up appointments because they moved or they just plain forgot. If these dropouts have a different prognosis, then you have trouble.

Who stopped or switched therapies? If there are compliance issues, handle the noncompliant patients carefully. Patients who have problems with compliance will also often have trouble with other self-care habits and thus be at greater risk for adverse outcomes. Excluding noncompliant patients can lead to some serious biases.

2.2   Who was excluded at the start of the study?

Researchers, trying to minimize variation, will use exclusion criteria to create more homogeneous groups. Ask yourself the question, 'How similar are my patients?' If it is difficult to extrapolate results from a very tightly controlled and homogeneous clinical trial to the variation of patients seen in your practice, then the research has limited value to you.

There is a tension between minimizing variation and maximizing generalizability (Godwin 2003; Siderowf 2004). The trials with minimal exclusion criteria are called pragmatic trials and are intended to measure effectiveness, the ability of a drug or therapy to work under very general conditions. Trials with stricter exclusion criteria develop a more narrowly drawn population that can measure efficacy, the ability of a drug or therapy to work under ideal conditions. Though efficacy is less compelling in the real world, you have to establish it before trying to demonstrate effectiveness under more general conditions.

There are three very common and very serious exclusions in medical research that deserve special attention: exclusion of elderly patients, exclusion of women, and exclusion of children.

2.2.1   Exclusion of elderly patients

If you are elderly, pat yourself on the back. Your demographic group drives the health care economy. You are, by far, the largest consumers of new medications and new therapies. Yet, far too often, these new medications and new therapies are tested on patients much younger (Bayer 2000).

There is a simple reason for this exclusion. When researchers design their experiments, they want a nice clean sample.

Researchers want patients who are ill with one and only one disease. But with older people, several things will break down at the same time (Schellevis 1993).

Researchers do not want patients who are taking a lot of other medications. But older people take so many different drugs that they often qualify for bulk discounts at the local drug store.

Finally, researchers want patients who are likely to stay alive for the duration of the research study. But older people are likely to die from conditions unrelated to disease being studied.

Although the reasons for excluding elderly patients are understandable, they are still not justifiable. Research done on younger patients cannot be easily generalized to older patients.

2.2.2   Exclusion of women

Several decades ago, there was a large study of aspirin as a primary prevention against heart attacks (Physicians Health Study Research Group 1989). This study recruited over 20,000 physicians and asked them to take either a small dose of aspirin or a placebo every day. They had to follow these physicians for five to ten years because they would not cooperate and have heart attacks faster. At the completion of the study, the researchers announced that aspirin was highly successful at preventing heart attacks.

There was one major problem with the research sample. Every single one of the physicians studied was male. Not a single female was included in the sample. It is not as though this was a problem only for men. Heart disease kills more women than any other condition.

There are some legitimate concerns when testing drugs that might harm a developing fetus, but you can handle this with careful restrictions to women who are not sexually active and/or who are using an effective form of birth control. In addition, some conditions, such as prostate cancer, cannot be tested in women.

There is some dispute over whether gender bias still exists, with one study arguing that it still occurs (Ramasubbu 2001) and another arguing it does not (Meinert 2001). When the exclusion of women occurs, it raises troubling questions and hinders your ability to generalize the results of the research.

2.2.3   Exclusion of children

At the opposite extreme from the elderly are children. This group, sadly, is also left out too often from the benefits of research.[1]

Children are not little adults. The liver in a child will process drugs quite differently from the liver of an adult. The nutritional demands of a growing child are quite different than those of a fully grown adult. And if you thought that your children became unpredictable as they went through puberty, try looking at them from a medical perspective!

---

[1] My supervisor, Ralph Kauffman, gave some excellent testimony about this before a Congressional subcommittee looking at FDA approval of drugs for children. You can read his comments at: www.aap.org/advocacy/washing/offlabel.htm.

No one wants to see our children used as guinea pigs, and there are special ethical reviews and safeguards that we must comply with when we study children.

Our failure, however, to study children in a careful controlled setting will end up subjecting all children to a large and uncontrolled experiment with no prospect of learning which treatments are safe for children and which ones are harmful.

2.2.4   Excluding troublemakers

A new trend in medical research is to treat all patients with a placebo for a short time and then exclude from the study anyone who responds too strongly to the placebo. The idea is that if you remove these patients from the sample, the response rate in the placebo group for the full study might be lower which increases the difference between the placebo group and the treatment group. This is a very active area of research, and there is some data to suggest that placebo responders differ in important ways from other patients (Leuchter 2002).

If this sounds like cheating, some people would agree with you. As a practicing clinician, you have no way of telling which patients would respond well to a placebo, and even if you did, you would not refuse to treat such patients. Furthermore, there is empirical evidence that excluding placebo responders does not enhance the apparent effectiveness of a treatment (Lee 2004).

Another purpose of the short term placebo administration to all patients is to see who is capable of meeting the informational demands and the logistical requirements of the research. Researchers will identify patients who cannot fill out a diary regularly or who are haphazard in their collection of data. These patients are dropped from the study before they can do any harm to the research.

There are both practical and ethical arguments against a preliminary evaluation of a placebo in all patients (Senn 1997; Evans 2000). The ethical concerns involve the intentional deception of the patient. Notice that this differs from a blinded study, in which you tell the patients that they will not know what treatment they receive until after the study is over. The patients know that you are intentionally withholding this information in order to improve the validity of the science, and if they are uncomfortable with this, they can refuse to participate in the research. An initial short term placebo evaluation differs markedly, since a doctor is hardly likely to say: 'Take this ineffective substance for the next month and record your symptoms daily in this diary' (Senn 1997).

From a practical perspective, you do not care whether a patient is sloppy in filling out a diary. You treat that patient the same as any other patient. More importantly, there may be reason to believe that patients who make lousy research subjects might have a worse prognosis than patients who are more meticulous. If this is true, excluding the troublemakers is like putting on a pair of rose-colored glasses.

2.2.5   Other important exclusions

Sometimes the exclusions in a research study are subtle. A commonly repeated story (although I am not sure if it is true or not) involves a researcher who compared the IQ scores of prisoners to those of the general public. Noting a large gap, the researcher concluded that criminals have lower IQs than honest people. This comparison, though, used a sample not of all criminals, but of those who got caught.

If you wanted to study adolescent drug use, you might consider a survey of high school students. This survey, though, would exclude anyone who dropped out of school. The dropouts have a far higher rate of drug usage than teenagers who stay in school. If you are interested in all adolescents, but your research design excludes dropouts, you will seriously underestimate drug use (Swaim 1997). In a different situation, of course, this might not be a terrible problem. It depends on your perspective. A principal trying to understand patterns of drug use in his/her high school, for example, might actually prefer to exclude dropouts.

A rather clever understanding of these subtle exclusions appeared in an article on selection bias (Wainer 1998) as well as on the famous American radio show, 'Car Talk'. The hosts of the 'Car Talk' program, Tom and Ray Magliozzi, offer a puzzle each week for their listeners. Most of the time it relates to auto mechanics, but this particular puzzle involved a nameless mathematician who was asked during World War II to help with a military problem.[2] A lot of bombers were not returning from their missions, so the Royal Air Force wanted to put armor on the bombers. But where to put it? They could not put it everywhere because the bomber would be so heavy that they could not take off. So this mathematician looked at the planes that returned and noted where they had holes from enemy fire. These holes were distributed more or less randomly throughout the plane except for two regions where there was nothing. His recommendation was to place the armor only in those two areas where no enemy fire was found. This seems counterintuitive, which is why it makes such a good puzzle.

This mathematician hypothesized that any plane hit in those regions did not survive to return. The other areas could be hit and the plane could still limp back to safety. This is an example of selection bias. The bombers in the

---

[2] You can read the original on the Car Talk websites, both the question (www.cartalk.com/content/puzzler/transcripts/199838/index.html) and the answer (www.cartalk.com/content/puzzler/transcripts/199839/answer.html).

study were not a random sample of all bombers; they were a sample of bombers that returned safely.

If you read the account in Wainer (1998), you will learn that the nameless mathematician was Abraham Wald. This article also has several other amusing examples of subtle and not-so-subtle exclusions, including research into the most dangerous occupation of all. An occupation where the average life expectancy is only 20.7 years. And what is this dangerous occupation? Student.

2.2.6   Exclusions: What to look for

Not all exclusions are bad. Here are some issues to consider:

- Are the excluded patients likely to have a worse prognosis?
- Are any major demographic groups left out or seriously underrepresented?
- Are any of the exclusion criteria artificial and unrepresentative of the patients that you normally see?

2.3   Who refused to join the study?

Quite often, the only patients we are able to study are those who volunteer to help out. The use of volunteers, however, may exclude important segments of the patient population.

Volunteers may differ from the normal population in several important ways. Volunteers for a study involving cash payments may come more often from economically challenged environments. If a free health checkup is included, volunteers may come more often from people worried about their health status. Volunteers for lengthy studies are less likely to be employed.

Smokers who volunteer for a smoking cessation study are quite different than smokers in general (Hughes 1997). It should be obvious, but sometimes it is easy to forget this important distinction. Sometimes you are interested in generalizing to all smokers and sometimes you are interested in generalizing to all smokers who are trying to quit.

2.3.1   Volunteers for painful procedures

Recruiting controls is especially troublesome in a study that involves a painful procedure. A Swedish study documents volunteer bias in a study of personality (Gustavsson 1997). In this study, the researchers wanted to analyze cerebrospinal fluid in order to 'examine the associations between personality traits and biochemical variables'.

Now, how do you get cerebrospinal fluid? The technical term is lumbar puncture, but it is also called a spinal tap. A spinal tap is rather painful, I am told, and it carries a small risk of some serious side effects. What sort of person would volunteer to submit to a spinal tap?

In this study, the subjects they recruited had already completed a complete personality profile in a previous research study. Of the 87 subjects, 48 declined to participate. There was one personality trait that was quite different between the 'volunteers' and the 'refusers'. Can you guess what it is?

It turns out that the volunteers had scores roughly a half standard deviation higher on impulsiveness. They did not differ on other personality traits such as socialization and detachment. The large difference in the impulsiveness measurement would obviously cloud any attempt to correlate personality traits and biochemical measurements in spinal fluids among those who volunteered.

2.3.2   Professional volunteers

Many drug companies pay good money for healthy volunteers to test new drugs. If the study involves extensive observation and/or invasive procedures, the amount of money offered can add up. Some volunteers will return repeatedly for different studies. No one gets rich this way, and the amount of money offered cannot be so large to be coercive. But serving as a research volunteer can still help pay a few bills and supplement your income.

Do these professional volunteers differ from you and me? You might suspect that these volunteers are poorer and less likely to have a full-time job. There are some subtle differences that are even more important.

Example: When genetic testing was done on a group of professional volunteers, there were almost no instances of a genetic variation that was associated with slow metabolism of certain drugs (Chen 1997). This slow metabolism would tend to be associated with a greater chance of side effects. This may not be too surprising. If you have a bad outcome with your first research study, you will probably not come back for the next study. Unfortunately, this means that studies on professional volunteers could possibly understate the likelihood and severity of side effects, as compared to the general population.

2.3.3   Nonresponse

An aspect of volunteering can occur in survey studies. People who volunteer to return a questionnaire are frequently quite different from those who refuse to fill out the survey. In particular, the nonresponders tend to be more apathetic. Return rates for surveys vary by the type of survey, but if less than half of the subjects returned the survey, any results are of very limited value. Again, look for efforts to minimize nonresponse and/or efforts to characterize the demographics of nonresponders.

Example: Two researchers examined general practitioners who routinely failed to return mail surveys (Stocks 2000). A follow-up telephone call assessed demographic characteristics of this group. They were older, less likely to have postgraduate qualifications, and less likely to be involved with a teaching practice.

Volunteer bias can be especially troublesome when you are examining issues that are considered by some people to be embarrassing or personal. Two American researchers examined the characteristics of people who were willing and unwilling to volunteer for studies about sexuality (Strassberg 1995). Volunteers had a more positive attitude towards sex, less guilt, and more sexual experiences.

2.3.4   Refusals: What to look for

Most studies use volunteers, so you cannot just pooh-pooh a study for this reason alone. Here are some questions you should ask:

- Are the incentives for participating related to important prognostic factors?
- What are the disincentives for participating? Are any of these important?
- Were the researchers able to characterize various aspects of those who did not volunteer? How similar were the volunteers and nonvolunteers?

2.4   Who stopped or switched therapies?

When you give a drug to your patients, unless you watch them as they swallow the pill, you have no guarantee that they took the drug. This is also true for most research studies. The research subjects may not comply with the demands of the study. They may take only some of the medication, may stop taking the medication entirely, or may even switch to the competing medicine. Issues involving compliance are difficult to handle and there is no perfect way to analyze these patients.

Problems with compliance will usually end up diluting the impact of the new therapy. At the extreme, if 100% of your patients are noncompliant in both arms of the study, then you will surely see no difference between any two drugs. Although I discuss compliance from the perspective of a drug study, it is also an issue in nondrug studies. If a patient fails to show up for therapy sessions, or forgoes a required operation, the same issues and problems as noncompliance with a drug regimen are raised.

2.4.1   Intention to treat

The intuitive approach is to remove from your study any patients who fail to comply with the protocol. This approach has its merits, but is generally avoided. What most researchers use instead is an 'intention to treat' (ITT) approach. With ITT, the patients are analyzed in the groups to which they were originally randomized regardless of how much or how little medication they have taken. In fact, if some of the patients have the opportunity to switch to the competing drug (or therapy) and do so, with ITT, you still analyze them as if they took the drug they were originally assigned to take.

There are several reasons why many researchers use ITT. First, researchers will often go to a lot of trouble to ensure randomized assignment in the study. Researchers in surgery have been known to take a sterilized coin into the operating room to choose which surgery to perform (Hollis 1999). When you go to such great lengths to use randomization, you do not want to abandon it without a fight. And when choices by the patient about whether they comply with the protocol start to determine who gets analyzed in which group, you lose randomization and all the benefits that it confers.

Second, with ITT, you get a more realistic picture of the new drug or therapy. If a drug or therapy is difficult to comply with, then that difficulty ought to be considered as part of the whole package. If noncompliance for a difficult-to-tolerate drug dilutes the impact of that drug, then it is worth knowing. Keep the noncompliant patients in because you will likely encounter the same patients among those whom you regularly treat.

Third, ITT can prevent some serious biases in the research. Consider a new surgical therapy which is being compared to a standard nonsurgical therapy. Some patients randomized to the surgical therapy might die before receiving the therapy. This is the most extreme form of noncompliance. These patients should still be analyzed as part of the surgical therapy group. Otherwise, the rapidly dying patients will be excluded from the treatment group, but not from the control group, leading to serious problems.

As a general rule, noncompliant patients will usually have worse outcomes than compliant patients. In fact, there is solid evidence that patients who fail to comply with a placebo have worse outcomes than patients who comply with a placebo (Coronary Drug Project Research Group 1980; Horwitz 1990). I was quite amazed when I first saw evidence of this, but it actually makes sense. Patients who comply poorly with a placebo probably have other poor self-care habits.

2.4.2   Intention to treat: What to look for

When you are looking at compliance issues, consider the following issues:

- Was any attempt made to assess compliance?
- Was the compliance level similar to patients seen in your practice?
- Would additional analysis, using the treatment actually received, answer a different, but still important question?

2.5   Who dropped out during the study?

It is inevitable that some patients will drop out during the study. If the number is more than a few, this is a cause for concern. Dropouts often have a different prognosis than those who stay. Ignoring the dropouts will often paint a rosier picture of the outcome. Was there any effort (financial inducement, follow-up reminders) made to minimize dropouts? Were the authors able to characterize the demographics of the dropouts?

2.5.1   Is the dropout caused by the treatment itself or a poor prognosis?

When the reason for dropping out is unrelated to the study, then you can ignore the dropouts without any serious problem. You lose a little bit of power and precision, but are otherwise okay.

If, on the other hand, dropping out is related to prognosis, be careful. If someone drops out of a cancer study to take laetrile treatments down in Mexico, that is often because the therapy assigned as part of the research is not working well.

You might be tempted to think that dropping out because of a move out of town is unrelated to prognosis. Often it is, but keep in mind that you will see more mobility among poorer patients. These patients will often have to move for economic reasons. So, if you leave these patients out, then you are excluding patients who are on the lower rungs of the socioeconomic ladder. These patients will often not do as well for a variety of reasons, and their loss will create a rosier and more optimistic sample than what you would encounter in the real world.

2.5.2   At what level should the number of dropouts be a concern?

There is no simple answer to this question. Smaller is better, of course, but there are no firm guidelines. I have seen some suggestions that if the rate is 10%, then dropouts are not a serious issue. There is no empirical justification for this value, but it seems reasonable enough to me. The larger the rate, the more chance for problems. A dropout rate of 50% or more is almost always a sign of serious problems.

2.5.3   Inferring outcomes for dropouts

Sometimes you can infer or impute a value for the patient who dropped out of the study.[3] All of these methods for inferring outcomes for dropouts are imperfect. While these approaches can sometimes compensate for a small number of dropouts, they cannot make a silk purse out of a sow's ear.

In some contexts, you can infer the status of dropouts as treatment failures. For example, if someone stops attending a smoking cessation program, you have fairly strong justification for treating such a patient as if they were smoking again. In a study of weight loss programs, dropouts could be assumed to have regained any weight that they may have lost. This is not a perfect assumption, but it should work well in practice.

If someone drops out part of the way through the study, one option is Last Observation Carried Forward. This option takes the intermediate outcome forward and treats it as the final outcome under the assumption that the final outcome would have been about the same (Mallinckrodt 2004). Another approach is to incorporate whatever information is available in a mixed model. In its simplest form, this model fits a trend line for each individual subject and pools those trend lines across groups of subjects. Those subjects with complete data contribute more to the estimate of time trends, but all subjects with one or more intermediate values will still contribute a limited amount of information.

There are several more sophisticated approaches for inferring outcomes for dropouts, hot deck imputation and multiple imputation. With hot deck imputation, you divide your data into relatively homogeneous subgroups. When you encounter a missing data value, select a random subject from the same homogeneous subgroup and substitute his/her value for the missing value. With multiple imputation, you infer a distribution for the outcome variable using information about the interrelationships between the outcome variable and other variables measured in the analysis. For patients

---

[3] An excellent introductory guide for inferring outcomes is on the Health Economics Resource Center website (www.herc.research.med.va.gov/FAQ_I9.htm).

with missing outcomes, a random value is selected from this inferred distribution. This creates a new data-set, which you analyze as usual. Now do this again five or ten more times. Each time, analyze your data. Now pool the results of these multiple analyses. Both of these approaches require a lot of work, but they have been proven to work well in practice.

Example: In a study of a quality of life measure, the AMC Linear Disability Score (Holman 2004), patients were asked to rate certain activities as either 'I could carry out the activity' or 'I could not carry out the activity.' But if the patient never had a chance to carry out a particular activity, they rated their response as not applicable. Guidance on how to handle the not applicable response varied from treating it as a negative response, or using an average of the responses on the other items in the score. These researchers showed that hot deck imputation performed better than these simplistic approaches.

2.5.4   Dropouts: What to look for

It would be a rare research study that had absolutely no dropouts, so you do not want to be too fussy.

- Is the proportion of patients who drop out large?
- Look for a description of who dropped out. Is this group different from those who completed the study?
- Can you infer something about the dropouts and impute a reasonable value for their outcome?

2.6   Counterpoint: Intention to treat is overrated

The demand for an intention to treat analysis has become almost reflexive in the research community. Authors of systematic overviews will often cite the failure to use an intention to treat analysis as a methodological flaw (e.g. Lawlor 2001).

Nevertheless, there is still a place for the analysis that excludes noncompliant patients. This analysis answers the question, what will happen if I prescribe this drug to a group of patients who all take the drug regularly? The ITT analysis answers a different question: what will happen if I prescribe this drug to a group of patients that includes both compliant and noncompliant patients? It may help know the answers to both questions.

Example: The MRFIT trial was a randomized comparison of a special intervention to usual care (Cutler 1991). The special intervention encouraged smoking cessation and dietary changes. A comparison of the groups as they were randomized represented a comparison of the special intervention itself.

A comparison of the groups that actually changed represented a different comparison, because some of the people in the special intervention ignored the advice while some of the people in the usual care group changed their habits on their own. This second comparison was of nonrandomized groups, since the patients themselves determined their group membership. Nevertheless, it was interesting, because it involved a comparison, not of the encouragement itself, but of the actual changes that were being encouraged.

Since noncompliant patients can cause so much trouble, one dubious approach that researchers take is not to let these noncompliant patients into the study at all. A placebo drug is given to all patients during a single blind run-in period, and anyone who does not comply with the placebo is excluded from the study. This is the same philosophy of excluding troublemakers discussed earlier and it has the exact same problems.

The intent of this exclusion seems good on the surface. Problems with compliance will tend to dilute the effectiveness of a new therapy. At the extreme of 0% compliance, there is no possible way to distinguish effectiveness. So excluding noncompliant patients before the study starts will avoid this dilution effect.

The problem is that the researchers have jumped from the frying pan of compliance problems into the fire of poor generalizability. Unlike the researchers, you do not have the option of only treating patients who are compliant. And you will not have any reasonable way to screen out those noncompliant patients for special handling. So excluding noncompliant patients causes the same problems as excluding children, women, or the elderly.

Example: In a study of allergy shots (Adkinson 1997), children with asthma were evaluated during a run-in phase that lasted an average of 400 days. This lengthy phase was intended to ensure stability of the disease. Patients were only included in full study only if they used asthma medications on a daily basis or bronchodilators five to seven days per week. The value of an asthma shot, however, is that you can ensure compliance because it is done in your office. So even though these shots were not demonstrated to be effective in a population of children who comply with their other medications, perhaps they might still be effective in a broader population of children that sometimes forget to take their pills on time.

2.7   Summary—Who was left out?

Exclusion of subjects can make the study biased or less generalizable.

Who was excluded at the start of the study? Excessively strict entry criteria in a research study can make it difficult to extrapolate to the types of patients that you normally see.

Who refused to join the study? Do the volunteers differ substantially from refusers in ways that might influence the outcome of the study?

Who stopped or switched therapies? If there are compliance issues, handle the noncompliant patients carefully.

Who dropped out during the study? Did these dropouts have a different prognosis?

2.8 On your own

1. Review the inclusion and exclusion criteria of the following study. The abstract and the relevant portions of the methods section are reproduced below:

The risk of menstrual abnormalities after tubal sterilization: a case-control study. Shobeiri, M.J. and Atashkhoii, S. *BMC Women's Health* 2005, 5(1): 5.

Abstract. Background: Tubal sterilization is the method of family planning most commonly used. The existence of the post-tubal-ligation syndrome of menstrual abnormalities has been the subject of debate for decades. **Methods:** In a cross-sectional study, 112 women with the history of Pomeroy type of tubal ligation achieved by minilaparotomy as the case group and 288 women with no previous tubal ligation as the control group were assessed for menstrual abnormalities. **Results:** Menstrual abnormalities were not significantly different between the case and control groups ($p = 0.824$). The abnormal uterine bleeding frequency differences in two different age groups (30–39 and 40–45 years old) were statistically significant ($p = 0.0176$). **Conclusion:** Tubal sterilization does not cause menstrual irregularities.

Methods. This cross-sectional case-control study has been carried out on 500 women at Al-zahra hospital during 1999–2001 to assess the effect of tubal sterilization on the menstrual cycle. 260 women with abnormal uterine bleeding referred for diagnostic curettage, and 240 healthy women under the coverage of the hospital family planning center were selected randomly, and all were assessed for tubal ligation.

All women aged 30–46 were selected from a low-income urban population, with body weight between 50 and 90 kg. In the abnormal uterine bleeding group, those who had intrauterine device (IUD), leiomyoma on sonography, uterine size of greater than 9 cm or suffered from medical disorders were excluded from the study. Of 260 patients with menstrual irregularities, 30 subjects were excluded from the study. From the remaining 230 subjects, assessed for tubal sterilization, 87 patients had tubal ligation. Of 240 healthy women assessed for tubal ligation, 95 had previous tubal ligation. Totally 182 subjects with previous tubal ligation (case) and

288 subjects with no history of previous tubal ligation (control) were compared for abnormal uterine bleeding. Those subjects in the case group who had menstrual abnormalities, IUD, medical disorders or were on hormonal contraception, during the first year prior to the sterilization were excluded from the study. Those who were at least 30 and at most 40 years of age by the time of tubal ligation and had Pomeroy type of interval tubal ligation via minilaparotomy were included in the study. Finally, considering the exclusion and inclusion criteria, 112 subjects remained in the case group and 288 with no tubal ligation in the control group were evaluated for menstrual abnormalities.

This is an open source publication. The full free text is available at www.biomedcentral.com/1472-6874/5/5.

2. Review the inclusion and exclusion criteria of the following study. The abstract and the relevant portions of the methods section are reproduced below:

Comparison of energy-restricted very low-carbohydrate and low-fat diets on weight loss and body composition in overweight men and women. Volek, J., Sharman, M., Gomez, A., Judelson, D., Rubin, M., Watson, G., Sokmen, B., Silvestre, R., French, D., and Kraemer, W. J. *Nutritional Metabolism* (Lond) 2004, 1(1): 13.

Abstract. Objective: To compare the effects of isocaloric, energy-restricted very low-carbohydrate ketogenic (VLCK) and low-fat (LF) diets on weight loss, body composition, trunk fat mass, and resting energy expenditure (REE) in overweight/obese men and women. **Design:** Randomized, balanced, two-diet period clinical intervention study. Subjects were prescribed two energy-restricted (500 kcal/day) diets: a VLCK diet with a goal to decrease carbohydrate levels below 10% of energy and induce ketosis and a LF diet with a goal similar to national recommendations (%carbohydrate:fat:protein=~60:25:15%). **Subjects:** 15 healthy, overweight/obese men (mean ± s.e.m.: age 33.2 ± 2.9 years, body mass 109.1 ± 4.6 kg, body mass index 34.1 ± 1.1 kg/m^2) and 13 premenopausal women (age 34.0 ± 2.4 y, body mass 76.3 ± 3.6 kg, body mass index 29.6 ± 1.1 kg/m^2). **Measurements:** Weight loss, body composition, trunk fat (by dual-energy X-ray absorptiometry), and resting energy expenditure (REE) were determined at baseline and after each diet intervention. Data were analyzed for between group differences considering the first diet phase only and within group differences considering the response to both diets within each person. **Results:** Actual nutrient intakes from food records during the VLCK (%carbohydrate:fat:protein=~9:63:28%) and the LF (~58:22:20%) were significantly different. Dietary energy was restricted, but was slightly higher during the VLCK (1855 kcal/day) compared to the LF (1562 kcal/day) diet for men. Both between and within group comparisons revealed a distinct advantage of a VLCK over a LF diet for weight loss, total fat loss, and trunk fat loss for men (despite significantly greater energy intake). The majority of women also responded more favorably to the VLCK diet, especially in terms of trunk fat loss. The greater reduction in trunk fat was not merely due to the greater total fat loss, because the ratio of trunk fat/total fat was also significantly reduced during the VLCK diet in men and women. Absolute REE (kcal/day) was decreased with both diets as expected, but REE expressed relative to body mass (kcal/kg), was better maintained on the VLCK diet for men only. Individual responses clearly show the majority of men and women experience greater weight and fat loss on a VLCK than a LF diet. **Conclusion:** This study shows a clear benefit of a VLCK over LF diet for short-term body weight and fat loss, especially in men. A preferential loss of fat in the trunk region with a VLCK diet is novel and potentially clinically significant but requires further validation. These data provide additional support for the concept of metabolic advantage with diets representing extremes in macronutrient distribution.

Methods. A total of 28 healthy volunteers (15 men and 13 women) were recruited by flyers and word-of-mouth. Subjects were between 20 and 55 years, nonsmokers, and greater than 25 % body fat determined via dual-energy X-ray absorptiometry (DEXA). Subjects went through a thorough screening procedure to ensure they would be committed to completing the study. Exclusion criteria included a body mass >145 kg (because of technical difficulties in performing DEXA), postmenopausal women, overt diabetes, cardiovascular, respiratory, gastrointestinal, thyroid or any other metabolic disease, weight change ± 2 kg over the last month, adherence to special diets, use of nutritional supplements (except a daily multivitamin/mineral), and use of medications to control blood lipids or glucose. The majority of subjects were sedentary and were instructed not to start an exercise program during the study. Those who were active were instructed to maintain the same level of physical activity throughout the study.

This is an open source publication. The full free text is available at www.nutritionandmetabolism.com/content/1/1/13.

3. Review the reasons listed for dropping out in the following study. Discuss to what extent do these dropouts compromise the integrity of the research study.

Participant characteristics associated with withdrawal from a large randomized trial of spermicide effectiveness. Raymond, E.G., Chen, P.L., Pierre-Louis, B., Luoto, J., Barnhart, K. T., Bradley, L., Creinin, M.D., Poindexter, A., Wan, L., Martens, M., Schenken, R., Nicholas, C. F., and Blackwell, R. *BMC Medical Research Methodology* 2004, 4(1): 23.

Background: In most recent large efficacy trials of barrier contraceptive methods, a high proportion of participants withdrew before the intended end of follow-up. The objective of this analysis was to explore characteristics of participants who failed to complete seven months of planned participation in a trial of spermicide efficacy. **Methods:** Trial participants were expected to use the assigned spermicide for contraception for 7 months or until pregnancy occurred. In bivariable and multivariable analyses, we assessed the associations between failure to complete the trial and 17 prespecified baseline characteristics. In addition, among women who participated for at least 6 weeks, we evaluated the relationships between failure to complete, various features of their first 6 weeks of experience with the spermicide, and characteristics of the study centers and population. **Results:** Of the 1,514 participants in this analysis, 635 (42%) failed to complete the study for reasons other than pregnancy. Women were significantly less likely to complete if they were younger or unmarried, had intercourse at least eight times per month, or were enrolled at a university center or at a center that enrolled fewer than four participants per month. Noncompliance with study procedures in the first 6 weeks was also associated with subsequent early withdrawal, but dissatisfaction with the spermicide was not. However, many participants without these risk factors withdrew early. **Conclusions:** Failure to complete is a major problem in barrier method trials that seriously compromises the interpretation of results. Targeting retention efforts at women at high risk for early withdrawal is not likely to address the problem sufficiently.

This is an open source publication. The full free text is available at: www.biomedcentral.com/1471-2288/4/23.

Mountain or Molehill? The Clinical Importance of the Results

3.1 Introduction

Do the research results add up to something important or are the results trivial? For the results to be important, the study needs to have a narrow focus, it has to measure the right outcomes, and the change in the outcome has to be large from a clinical perspective.

3.1.1 Case study: Side effects of vaccination

A pair of articles on vaccination that appeared next to each other in a 1999 issue of *British Medical Journal* (Karvonen 1999; Henderson 1999) offer an interesting contrast in reporting styles. I commented about this on the *BMJ* webpages (Simon 1999).

Both studies used a cohort design to examine side effects of vaccination. In the first article, the authors compared the rate of Type I diabetes among children vaccinated with *Haemophilus influenzae* type b at the age of 3 months to children vaccinated at the age of 24 months. They reported the relative risk as 1.06 ($p = 0.54$). In the second study, the authors compared the risk of intermittent wheezing between children with and without pertussis vaccine. They also reported the relative risk as 1.06 (95% CI: 0.81–1.37).

Both studies are negative, but the second study tells you something extra. In that study, you know that even after allowing for sampling error, there is no justification for believing that the risk of side effects could be increased by 50%. You know this because the relative risk of 1.5 lies outside the confidence interval. With the first study, you are left wondering: this looks like a small relative risk, but is it possible that sampling error would allow for a 50% or 100% increase in risk? You would have to calculate the confidence interval for yourself to be sure.

Since you have been such a good reader, I shall save you the trouble. The 95% confidence interval for the relative risk in the first study is 0.88–1.28. So you can rule out a large change in risk in this study as well.

Unfortunately, neither study reported a measure of absolute risk. With a bit of effort, you can calculate these values yourself. In the first study, the number needed to harm for Type I diabetes is 4,500 (95% CI: 1,100 to infinity). You would expect one case of diabetes for every 4,500 children vaccinated. In the second study, the number needed to harm for intermittent wheezing is 109 (95% CI: 37 to infinity). You would expect one case of intermittent wheezing for every 109 children vaccinated.

These calculations are important. You need to know what the best course of action is with respect to these vaccinations. If there is a large risk that outweighs the benefit of the vaccination, you should stop vaccinating your patients. Even if the risk does not outweigh the benefit, if it is large enough, you should warn people about the side-effect risk.

Notice that I did not define 'large' here. How much of an increase in side-effect risk is large? It is an easier question to ask than to answer, but in the case of vaccines, the answer is especially difficult. What disease is the vaccine trying to prevent? How much more prevalent would that disease become if people stopped using the vaccine? Is the disease life threatening? How serious is the side effect?

These are complicated questions, but they are questions that you have to ask if you want to assess whether the research findings add up to a mountain or if they are just an unimportant molehill.

3.1.2   Mountain or molehill? What to look for

Make sure that any research study measures something of practical importance.

Did they measure the right thing? Researchers should focus on outcomes of interest to the patient and long-term rather than short-term outcomes. Examining multiple outcome measures or multiple subgroups will dilute the quality and strength of the evidence.

Did they measure it well? Certain types of measurements have a lower strength of evidence. Be cautious about measurements that are retrospective because memory is imperfect. Unblinded measurements can allow your patients' expectations to influence the outcome. Do not trust unvalidated/ unreliable measurements or *post hoc* changes in the protocol.

Were the changes clinically important? With a large enough sample size, a difference between two groups that is statistically significant might represent a change so small as to be clinically trivial. Specify a clinically important change for a study by asking how much of a change would be needed to convince you to adopt a new treatment or therapy. For negative trials, look for a precise confidence interval or a justification of the sample size that was conducted before data collection.

3.2   Did they measure the right thing?

There is a well-known story about a man who was fumbling about in the middle of the street on a very dark night. A passerby stopped and asked what was going on. The man replied, 'I dropped my keys and I can't find them'. So the passerby agrees to help look for the lost keys. After a half hour, the passerby gets frustrated and asks the man if he remembers exactly where he was standing when he dropped the keys. 'Over in the alley there' came the response. The passerby looked with surprise and exasperation at the man. 'Over in the alley? Then why are you looking out here in the middle of the street?' The man replied, 'Because the light is better here.'

3.2.1   Surrogate Measures

Patients are generally interested in one of four things. Mortality (will I die?), morbidity (will I go blind?), symptoms (will I throw up?), or quality of life (will I be able to walk up a flight of steps without getting winded?). They do not care about concentration of homocysteine in their blood or what their CD4 cell count is unless those values relate to something that is important to them.

Good research, then, should measure something that is important to patient. There is an acronym for this, POEM, which stands for Patient Oriented Evidence that Matters (www.infopoems.com). Every research study should directly measure an outcome that matters to the patient. Direct measurements, though, are often difficult to obtain. So sometimes researchers will examine intermediate measures that are faster and easier to assess, but which may or may not be predictive of more important end points. These intermediate measures are called surrogate measures.

Some examples of surrogate measures are forced expiratory volume and premature ventricular contractions. These measures are not important to a patient in themselves, but only in their ability to translate into events that patients care about. Does an improvement in forced expiratory volume translate into a reduction in asthma attacks? Does a reduction in abnormal ventricular depolarization translate into a reduction in the recurrence of heart attacks?

You have to show a strong relationship between the surrogate measure and the patient-oriented outcome. If there is only a weak relationship, then establishing a large effect on the surrogate measure will not translate into a large effect on the patient-oriented outcome.

You also need to establish that changes in the surrogate measure lead to changes in the outcome of interest. The surrogate measure might be strongly correlated with the patient-oriented outcome but only because both are related to a third factor. That third factor might end up being the measure that you need to change, not the surrogate measure.

You also need to assure yourself that the surrogate measure is sensitive to changes associated with improvement in health. There are a wide range of measures of pulmonary function, for example, and some are more responsive than others to changes in health (de Torres 2002).

Example: A study that showed an association between duration of breastfeeding and brachial artery distensibility at 20–28 years of age (Leeson 2001) recognized that brachial artery distensibility is a surrogate outcome. Distensibility is a measure of stiffness, and could be considered a marker for cardiovascular disease in later life. Such a link is tenuous and the authors themselves, as well as an accompanying editorial (Booth 2001), admit that this does not establish a cause-and-effect relationship between breastfeeding and heart disease.

Example: A study of chemotherapy for colorectal cancer (Buyse 2000) noted that tumor response was often used to assess the value of new treatments, but there was an uncertain connection between tumor response and mortality. The authors demonstrated through a meta-analysis that there was a link between tumor response and survival, but this link was weak. A 50% improvement in tumor response would only lead to a 6% change in the odds of death.

Example: A study of cholesterol lowering drugs (Law 2003), showed a significant decrease in LDL cholesterol and, in contrast to the previous example, tied that lowering to a decreased risk of heart attacks and strokes. A 1.8 mmol/l change for example, was achieved and could be linked to a 61% reduction in the risk of ischemic heart disease and a 17% reduction in the risk of stroke.

3.2.2   Short-term changes in outcome

Perhaps it is just human nature, but we are all impatient and we want to focus on the short term and the immediate. That is true for researchers also. They want to do the research, publish it, and move on as quickly as possible. Using a short-term outcome measure facilitates this way of life. I am sure that budgetary constraints have something to do with this as well.

The problem with the focus on short-term outcomes is that it is usually easier to get a short-term change, but that is not what is really important from a clinical perspective. It is easy, for example, to get a smoker to quit smoking for a day, or maybe even a week. But most interventions that try to help people quit smoking do not work as well for keeping people off cigarettes for three months or for two years. Pretty much any diet works well in the first week or so. People will lose a few pounds right away. But can people continue to lose weight and maintain that weight loss for a full year? That is a much harsher but much more realistic test of the value of a diet.

Example: A study of a youth tobacco education program (Mahoney 2002) looked at immediate recall and recall four months later about the knowledge and attitudes that this program was trying to reinforce. Although most concepts were retained for the short term, only two were retained at the four-month evaluation: 'recognition that smokers have yellow teeth and fingers' and 'smoking one pack of cigarettes a day costs several hundred dollars per year.'

3.2.3   Multiple outcome measures

The presence of a narrowly drawn research plan developed before the start of data collection adds a great deal to the credibility of a study. In contrast, a scattershot approach will dilute the credibility of the research. There is a saying in Statistics circles, 'If you torture your data long enough, it will confess to something.'

Example: A study of the relationship between childhood cancer and diet (Sarasua 1994) examined five different types of meat consumption (ham/bacon/sausage, hot dogs, hamburgers, lunch meats, and charcoal-broiled foods), two different types of cancer (acute lymphocytic leukemia and brain tumor), and considered the diet both of the child and of the mother during pregnancy. This led to 20 different combinations of these factors. In addition, the authors provided additional discussion using a different definition of high and low consumption. High consumption of hot dogs, for example, was defined as one or more hot dogs per week, but later results defining high consumption as two or more hot dogs were described.

A good research study has limited objectives that are specified in advance. There is solid empirical evidence that specifying a hypothesis before data collection reduced the chances of a false positive finding by a factor of 3 (Swaen 2001). Failure to limit the scope of a study leads to problems with multiple testing.

There are good reasons to look at multiple outcomes when you are trying to explore a new area. The results of this exploratory analysis would then provide justification and focus for a second study that would replicate the results. Looking at multiple outcomes is also fine if there are several distinct dimensions, like efficacy and side effects, that need to be evaluated. But looking at multiple outcome measures just because you can leads to a 'fishing expedition'—a study that looks at a large number of exposures or a large number of outcomes without any effort to prioritize.

Consider a hypothetical example of a drug company comparing their new pain relief drug to another company's drug. When they design the study, they look at pain levels every hour for five hours after the patient takes the drug. The multiple time points give the drug company extra chances to declare success (see Figures 3.1 and 3.2).

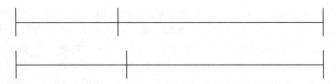

Figure 3.1. If the new drug shows a greater degree of relief earlier on in time, but a comparable amount of relief later, then they can claim that their product is faster acting.

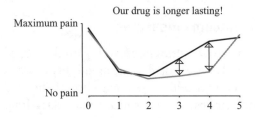

Figure 3.2. If the new drug shows a comparable degree of relief earlier, but a greater degree of relief later, then they can claim that their product is longer lasting.

There are statistical adjustments that you can use when you have multiple outcome measures. The simplest of these is called a Bonferroni correction. With the Bonferroni correction, you multiply the p-value for each outcome by the number of outcomes and see which ones are still smaller than the alpha level (usually 0.05). Equivalently, you could replace the alpha level of 0.05 with a value of 0.05 divided by the number of outcome measures. By making the threshold for any individual test so strict, the Bonferroni correction assures that the probability of making a Type I error for all of the outcome measures simultaneously is small. Researchers will often refer to a global null hypothesis: the hypothesis that none of the outcome measures differ between the treatment and control groups.

Example: In a study of personality traits (Kaasinen 2001), 61 patients with Parkinson's disease were compared to 45 age-matched controls. All subjects filled out the Temperament and Character Inventory (TCI) and the Karolinska Scales of Personality (KSP). The TCI scale measures novelty seeking, harm avoidance, reward dependence, self-directedness, cooperativeness, self-transcendence, and persistence. The KSP scale measures somatic anxiety, psychic anxiety, psychasthenia, inhibition of aggression, muscular tension, impulsiveness, monotony avoidance, detachment, socialization, social desirability, suspicion, guilt, indirect aggression, verbal aggression, and irritability. This is a total of 22 outcome measures, so the researchers compared each p-value to $0.05/22 = 0.00227$.

The Bonferroni comparison is quite controversial (Perneger 1998; Feise 2002) because it greatly increases the chances of a Type II error. Critics also claim that a global null hypothesis is rarely of direct interest. A possible compromise that I like is to compute both the regular p-value and a Bonferroni adjustment to the p-value. If both are significant, you have a strong positive finding. If neither is significant, you have a strong negative finding. If the regular p-value is significant, but the Bonferroni adjustment is not, then you have an 'interesting' finding that needs replication or corroboration from other sources.

3.2.4   Subgroup comparisons

Examining a large number of subgroups will dilute the credibility of a study. Maybe a drug is ineffective overall, but could you please check to see if it is effective in women? In patients with the most severe conditions? In patients younger than 30? In patients who smoke cigars? In patients who have a college education? In patients who live with a dog or cat? In patients who get a moderate amount of exercise?

Example: A light-hearted study on astrology (Pollex 2001) shows the problem with subgroup analysis. The researchers established a statistically significant association between certain astrological signs and winning the Nobel prize (Geminis were more likely; Leos were less likely). The authors conclude that 'foraging through databases using contrived study designs in the absence of biological mechanistic data sometimes yields spurious results'.

Subgroup comparisons suffer from three problems. First, the subgroup comparison is usually a nonrandomized comparison. Second, the subgroup comparison has less precision because the sample size is smaller. Third, the sample size in a study could be swamped by the potential number of possible subgroups that could potentially be examined.

If you find a subgroup that behaves differently, then you need to ask yourself a few questions. Is this a subgroup that I would have studied a priori if I had been more careful during the planning stage? Is there a plausible mechanism to explain why this subgroup behaves differently? Are there other studies that have similar findings for this subgroup?

Example: In a study of aspirin as a primary prevention against heart attacks (Meade 2000), the overall relative risk for coronary events was 0.80 showing a small protective effect of aspirin versus placebo. The effect, however, was far stronger (0.55 compared to 0.94) in patients with low systolic blood pressure (< 130 mm Hg) at entry compared to patients with higher pressures (>145 mm Hg). The authors were cautious about this finding, but argued that it was still credible because of the biological plausibility behind this particular subgroup.

There are some technical issues with subgroup comparisons. You would not want to declare that a therapy is effective for one subgroup if the p-value for that subgroup was 0.043 and the p-value for everyone else was 0.062. The analysis of subgroups should be done as a formal test of interaction.

3.2.5   Measuring the right outcome—What to look for

When you are looking at the outcome measured in a study, ask yourself the following questions:

- Is the outcome evaluating only short-term changes?
- Is the outcome related to an event that patients care about?
- Is the research diluted through the look at multiple outcomes or multiple subgroups?

3.3   Did they measure the outcome well?

Quality measurements are important for all variables, but they are especially important for the outcome measure. There are several types of measurements that provide weaker evidence. Be cautious about measurements that are retrospective, unblinded, self-reported, unvalidated, or unreliable.

3.3.1   Retrospective measurements

Retrospective measurements have less credibility than measurements taken prospectively. Retrospective data are those collected by looking backwards in time. We obtain this data by asking subjects to recall events that occurred earlier in their lives. We also get retrospective data when we review medical records, birth certificates, death certificates, or other sources of historical data. In contrast, data collected during the course of the study is known as prospective data.

Retrospective data are often inexpensive to collect, but you should be concerned about their accuracy. Historical data are often incomplete and it is sometimes difficult to verify their accuracy (Horwitz 1984). Therefore, retrospective data are considered less authoritative than prospective data.

The ability of a subject to recall information is sometimes affected by which group that they are in. Patients who experience a traumatic event (e.g. a cancer diagnosis or miscarriage) are more likely to search for and remember events that they feel might 'explain' this event, much more so than a group of comparable control subjects. It is not that they make up things, but rather that the control subjects do not have such a heightened level of awareness and will fail to recall things as well. This differential level of reporting is known as recall bias.

Example: In a study of self-reported pollution levels (Hunter 2004), 3,402 households were asked to characterize the pollution levels where they live. Respondents who had a person at home with respiratory symptoms were more likely to report poor air quality. This could possibly be a real effect of pollution or it might represent the heightened sensitivity to pollution for these households.

Another difficulty with retrospective data is that you may not be able to identify which was the cause and which was the effect. Causes have to occur before while effects have to occur after. But when you examine causes and effects retrospectively, you may end up losing information about timing.

There is an old joke about a statistician who was examining the fire department records, including information about how much damage the fire caused, and how many fire engines responded to the blaze. The statistician noticed a strong relationship between the two variables and concluded that the more fire engines you send, the more damage they cause.

Example: The *British Medical Journal* highlighted a research study where speech patterns were recorded in two groups of surgeons. The first group had two or more malpractice claims filed against them and the second group had none. There was a large difference between the two groups, with the first group having a dominant tone with less concern for the patient. The news report of this research suggested that: 'dominance coupled with a lack of anxiety in the voice may imply surgeon indifference and lead a patient to launch a malpractice suit when poor outcomes occur' (bmj.com/cgi/content/full/325/7359/297/a).

One reader, however, pointed out that perhaps 'being sued is a brutalizing and demoralizing experience and that this experience fundamentally changes the attitude of doctors towards their patients' (bmj.com/cgi/eletters/325/7359/297/a#24658).

Sometimes, though, you can establish credibility for retrospective measures. A review of research on smoking illustrates this well (Gail 1996). The author recalls a 1950 study that looked at the smoking habits of lung cancer patients and controls. The authors were concerned about the retrospective assessment of smoking among patients in both groups. Would patients with lung cancer exaggerate the amount of smoking? Would the interviewers press harder for information about smoking among the cancer patients? While it would be impossible to totally rule out recall bias, the authors did examine a third group, patients who were diagnosed with lung cancer and who later found out that they suffered from a different disease (false cases). If recall bias was the sole explanation of the difference in reported smoking, then the group of false cases should have had a similar level of smoking with the lung cancer patients. Instead they reported a lower level of smoking. This helped rule out the possibility that recall bias alone accounted for the higher reported smoking levels in the lung cancer patients.

3.3.2 Unblinded measurements

In an experimental study, it is desirable (but not always possible) to keep the information about the treatments hidden from the patients and from anyone involved with evaluating the patient. This is known as 'blinding' or 'masking'.Blinding prevents conscious or subconscious biases or expectations from influencing the outcome of the study.

Two researchers have examined studies with and without blinding. These authors found that studies without blinding show an average bias of 11–17% (Schulz 1996; Colditz 1989). In other words, when an unblinded study was compared to a blinded study, the former study tended to estimate a treatment effect that was (on average) 11–17% higher than the latter.

Additional evidence of this problem appears in a meta-analysis of the effect of intermittent sunlight exposure and melanoma (Nelemans 1995). When nine studies without blinding were combined, they showed an odds ratio of 1.84 which was statistically significant (95% confidence interval 1.52–2.25). When the seven studies with blinding were combined, they showed a much smaller odds ratio (1.17, 95% confidence interval 0.98–1.39), which was not statistically significant. This is further evidence that unblinded studies are more likely to show statistical significance than blinded studies.

There is always some individual who knows which patients get which treatments, such as the pharmacy that prepares the pills and placebos. This is perfectly fine as long as these individuals do not interact with the patients or evaluate the patients.

There is a bit of ambiguity with respect to who is blinded (Devereaux 2001). For example, a survey of 25 textbooks produced nine different definitions of 'double blind'. Therefore, you should avoid using these terms and focus instead on which individuals are blinded. If you are evaluating an article, look for evidence of blinding for the following groups:

- the patients themselves;
- clinicians who have substantial interactions with the patients;
- anyone who assesses outcomes in these patients; or
- anyone who collects data from these patients.

If only some of the above are unaware of the treatment, then the study is partially blinded.

Example: In a study of treatment for cerebral malaria (Aceng 2005), 103 children received either rectal artemether suppogels or a rectal placebo. The nurses administering the treatment knew which was the placebo, so this study was described as a single blind.

Blinding prevents the placebo effect from distorting the research results. The placebo effect is a product of 'belief, expectancy, cognitive reinterpretation, and diversion of attention' that can lead to psychological and sometimes physiological improvements in situations where the treatment is known to have no effect, such as sugar pills (Beyerstein 1997).

There are three specific situations where the placebo effect is of particular concern: when enthusiasm by the patient or the doctor for the new procedure is strong, when outcomes are based on the patient's self-assessment (e.g. quality of life studies), and when the treatment is primarily for symptoms (Johnson 1997). The placebo effect is less critical for objective outcomes like survival.

Even without a placebo effect, blinding would still be important to ensure uniform rates of compliance. You want to avoid a situation where a patient thinks 'I'm in the placebo arm, so it's not really important whether I show up for my follow-up evaluation.'

The value of blinding also extends to the research team, and should include anyone who interacts with the patients. In a clinical trial of treatments for multiple sclerosis, a pair of neurologists assessed the outcome of each patient (Noseworthy 1994). One neurologist was blinded to the treatment status and one was unblinded. The unblinded neurologist gave substantially lower ratings to patients in the placebo group, which would have led to falsely concluding that one of the treatments was effective.

Researchers can also influence the outcome in unblinded research through their attitudes and through their differential use of other medications (Schulz 2002).

Surgical procedures are often difficult to completely blind. Nevertheless, you can take some partial steps at blinding that prevent some of the biases from creeping in (Johnson 1997). If two surgical procedures use different types of incisions, identical blood or iodine stained opaque dressings could be used to keep the patients unaware of which operation was performed. Although the surgeon cannot be blinded to the difference in surgery, those who evaluate the health of the patient after surgery could be kept unaware of the particular operation, so as to ensure that their evaluation of the patient is unbiased.

Even though the placebo may look the same, sometimes the doctor may infer which group a patient belongs to, perhaps through noting a characteristic set of side effects for the active drug. Certain vitamins, for example, will turn your skin orange. If you are worried about side effects ruining the blind, ask the doctors to try to identify which treatment group they believe each patient belonged to. If the percentage of correct guesses is significantly larger than 50%, then the allocation scheme was not sufficiently blinded.

3.3.3 Self-report measurements

Self-report measurements, when the patients evaluate themselves, raise some special concerns. Patients often do not provide accurate assessments of their own helath.

Example: A comparison of self-report versus hospital records of resource utilization, (Kennedy 2002) showed substantial disagreement between the two measures, with individuals reporting substantially more use of physiotherapy than the hospital records would indicate.

Example: In a study of stress (Macleod 2002), there was a relationship between high levels of stress and increased rates for self-reported angina. There was no relationship, however, with more objective measures of heart disease. The apparent relationship with self-reported angina might be a tendency for some patients to overreport negative events (both psychological and medical) and for other patients to underreport negative events.

The degree to which patients report problems, for example, is associated with their level of education, as more educated patients are better able to describe their illnesses (Sen 2002).

You can only get certain measurements, such as pain, through self-report. Other measures, like quality of life, are best obtained directly from the patient (Moinpour 2000). Even when self-reported data is known to be inaccurate, there may still be substantial value in collecting it. The patient's perception of illness is always important, because health cannot be entirely reduced to objective numerical measures. After all, if you fix a patient's problem, but they leave your office thinking they are still ill, then you have a problem.

3.3.4   Measurements without established validity

Validity is a term that every discipline has a different definition for. In very simple and general terms, validity means that an outcome is measuring what you think it is measuring. There are several ways to measure validity, but most of these involve comparison to an external standard.

Example: A study of concussions (Piland 2003) used a 16-item self-reported scale and validated it by comparing it to composite balance and neuropsychological measures.

Example: In a validation study of motion palpation (Humphreys 2004), 20 chiropractic students were asked to identify the most hypomobile segment of the spine in patients with fused vertebrae. If the students failed to consistently identify the correct location in the extreme situation of a fused spine, their ability to diagnose more subtle spinal motion problems would be called into question. The students showed good levels of agreement with the location of the fused spine.

Example: In a study of methods to assess urine specific gravity (Steumpfle 2003), hydrometry and reagent strips showed consistent disagreements with refractometer measurements, and these methods could not be recommended for determining urine specific gravity measures during weight certification of collegiate wrestlers.

The classic example of a measurement without established validity is the Rorschach Ink Blot test. In this test, patients would be asked to interpret geometric figures that were essentially random and featureless forms. The interpretation given by the patient would reveal to a trained psychologist many insights into the patient's personality.

The ink blot test is difficult to evaluate under objective conditions, but when careful evaluations have been done, they have shown that this test has very limited ability to diagnose personality traits. It does have some ability to distinguish schizophrenic patients, but most of the other uses of this test have been discredited (Lilienfeld 2001).

Contrast this with the visual analog scale assessment of pain. To validate this measure, researchers examined how patients rated their pain before an operation and afterwards. They examined ratings before administration of analgesics and afterwards. When the scale showed changes under these conditions, it established the validity of the scale.

Be cautious about results that explain the role of race/ethnicity data in predicting a medical outcome (Walsh 2003). Quite often, race/ethnicity is not directly related to the outcome, but rather it is socioeconomic markers that are associated with race.

3.3.5   Measurements without established reliability

Reliability means different things in different fields, but the general concept is that a reliable measurement is one that would stay about the same if it were repeated under similar circumstances. Depending on the context, you would establish reliability differently. For example, one way to establish reliability is to have two people make independent assessments and show a good level of agreement. If you are measuring something that is stable over time, then you could take two measurements on different days or weeks and see how well they agree.

Example: In a study of range of motion (de Winter 2004), patients with shoulder pain were evaluated by two physical therapists using a digital inclinometer. The difference between the two raters had a standard deviation of 19.6 degrees for glenohumeral abduction and 18.8 degrees for external rotation. Both standard deviations are far larger than an amount of discrepancy considered acceptable (10 degrees or less). This indicates that measurements by different therapists would have poor reliability.

Be especially careful about measurements that have some level of subjectivity. If there is no establishment of reliability for these measures, then you have no assurance that the research is repeatable.

Wallace Sampson criticizes a study of homeopathic treatment for diarrhea (Jacobs 1994) because the outcome measures were all subjective measurements. The number of bowel movements, for example, as well as the smell and appearance of the feces, are open to interpretation. One could imagine first-time parents overreacting to small changes and being more likely to report that their child has diarrhea.

3.3.6 *Post hoc* changes

No research plan is perfect, and you should expect minor deviations from the plan in just about any research study. Major deviations, however, from the protocol can reduce the credibility of a study. Some examples of deviations from the plan include:

- investigating end points other than those originally specified;
- developing new exclusion criteria after the study has started; and
- stopping the study unexpectedly or extending it beyond the planned sample size.

You need to ask yourself if the authors deviated from the protocol in a conscious or subconscious effort to manipulate the results. Did the authors add other end points in order to salvage a largely negative study? Were new exclusion criteria targeted to keep 'troublesome' subjects out? It is impossible, of course, to discern the motives of the researchers. Nevertheless, for any deviation or modification to the protocol, you can ask whether this change would have made sense to include in the protocol if it had been thought of before data collection began.

Changes to the planned end of the study, either stopping the study early, or extending it beyond the planned sample size, can raise some serious problems (Ludbrook 2003). There are several reasons that you might want to stop a study early:

- early evidence that one of therapies is much better than the other (efficacy);
- early evidence that continuing the study would be unlikely to yield a significant result (futility);
- early evidence that one of the therapies is too dangerous (safety); and/or
- finishing the study would end up being far more expensive or time consuming than the original plan (economics).

Example: A study of fascial interposition during vasectomy (Sokal 2004) planned for an interim analysis halfway through the study. At that evaluation, patients randomized to receive fascial interposition had a much shorter time to azospermia and half the failure rate of the control group. These differences were so large that the study was halted early.

Example: A study of lung reduction surgery for patients with emphysema (The National Emphysema Treatment Trial Research Group 2001) ended the study early for a subgroup of patients with who have a low FEV1 and either homogeneous emphysema or a very low carbon monoxide diffusing capacity. In these patients, surgery had a 30-day mortality of 16% compared to 0% in the nonsurgical intervention group.

In order to maintain credibility, a study should have rules for stopping early that are specified before the start of data collection. Predetermined rules are especially important when a study ends early for efficacy. If a study ends early for economic reasons, and the result is not statistically significant, you need some assurance that the truncated sample size still provides a reasonable level of precision. In this situation, the width of the confidence intervals would indicate clearly whether the sample size was still adequate.

Extending a study beyond the original end date can also be problematic. Extensions for economic reasons (the budget went further than expected or an extra funding source appeared) is probably not a serious problem, but be very careful if the study gets extended because of a failure to achieve statistical significance at the planned sample size. The provisions for such an extension must be specified before the start of data collection.

3.3.7   Measuring the outcome well—What to look for

When you are looking at how the outcome was measured, ask yourself the following questions:

- Was the outcome dependent on the memory of the patients?
- Did the outcome have established validity and reliability?
- Were there *post hoc* changes in the protocol?

3.4   Were the changes clinically important?

Many journal authors have the bad habit of looking just at the *p*-value of a study and ignoring everything else. It is like there is a switch inside their brain that turns off the moment the *p*-value is calculated. Statistical significance, as measured by the *p*-value, is indeed important, but just as important is the clinical significance of the research.

It is difficult for me to talk about clinical importance because I am an outsider when it comes to medicine. I tell a story in my classes about how statisticians may be good with numbers but often have no perspective on their practical or clinical application.[1] A statistician is driving through the countryside in a beat-up old pick-up truck. He stops on the road to let a large flock of sheep pass. He calls out to the shepherd from the truck and brags that he can count the number of sheep in the flock to an accuracy of plus or minus five. The shepherd scoffs and offers a bet. 'If you can count the sheep that accurately, you can take one of the sheep home with you. If you are wrong, I get your pick-up truck'. The statistician agrees to the bet. After scanning the flock for a few seconds, he says that there are 527 sheep in the flock. The shepherd is dumbfounded. 'That's amazing', he says. 'You

---

[1] Again, I cannot take credit for this one. There are various forms of this joke on: www.bordercollierescue.org/breed_advice/ WorkingSheepdog.html.

were only off by one. Come on out and take any sheep you want'. So the statistician gets out and claims his prize. 'Wait', cries the shepherd, 'I'll bet you double or nothing that I can tell you what your day job is'. The statistician thinks this is a safe bet and agrees. The shepherd says, 'you are obviously a statistician'. Now the statistician is dumbfounded. 'How did you know?', he asks. 'Well', replies the shepherd, 'put down my sheepdog and I'll explain it to you'.

3.4.1   What exactly does clinical importance mean?

The pivotal word here is 'clinical'. To establish clinical importance, you need to use clinical judgment. I am not a clinician, so I cannot exercise clinical judgment. What I can do is get you to ask the right questions about clinical importance.

For a change to be clinically important, it has to be large enough for you to justify all the added trouble, expense, inconvenience, etc., to justify changing your clinical practice. You need to assess the size of the benefit relative to the cost of the treatment and the possible harms that might come from side effects.

You should incorporate your patient's values in this calculation, of course. Suppose that a drug has a side effect in that it reduces the fertility potential in the men who take it. For some men, no benefit is large enough if the treatment seriously hampers their ability to father a child. Other men might be indifferent to this side effect, and some might even consider it an added bonus.

David Sackett talks about 'particularizing' a research finding. If your patient belongs to a particular subgroup where the disease is more prevalent, or more virulent, or that subgroup is more likely to experience side effects, then you should adjust the research findings to fit the results of that subgroup. The calculations vary from situation to situation, but there are some good examples of particularizing them (see Ola 2001; Glasziou 1998).

There are some data to suggest that doctors and patients do not agree on the balance between benefits of a treatment relative to its costs and possible side effects. For example, when researchers interviewed 72 family physicians and 74 patients with hypertension (McAlister 2000), the patients were less likely to want antihypertensive treatments under conditions where doctors would normally encourage their use.

Not surprisingly, patients may not agree with themselves about clinical importance, nor should they. In a study of patients with artial fibrillation who might be candidates for warfarin therapy (Howitt 1999), one group of patients felt that warfarin would be worthwhile if their annual risk of stroke was at least 2.4%, while another group demanded a much higher average annual rate (4.1%) before they would adopt warfarin. The former group represented patients who had already adopted warfarin and the latter group represented patients who had refused warfarin treatment. I cannot say for sure what level of risk would justify warfarin therapy, of course, but I take some solace in the fact that these patients appeared to make choices consistent with their articulated beliefs.

3.4.2 Researchers will not define clinical importance for you

In a perfect world, the researchers would tell you how much of a change is important from a clinical perspective. After all, they are the experts in the area, or they would not be doing the research. Surprisingly, researchers are very reluctant to share this information (Chan 2001). Perhaps they have never thought of the issue in terms of clinical importance before. Perhaps they do not want to impose their values on the readers, or they do not want to commit to a particular viewpoint or perspective. Researchers may be uncomfortable doing this, but they should still offer an opinion. Even if you have a different perspective, when the researchers offer up an assessment of what they consider clinically important, it opens up the debate. It gets you thinking along the lines of 'is that the sort of difference that I would hope to see, or would I demand to see a larger difference instead?'

Example: In a study comparing two allergy drugs (Hampel 2003), a particular drug was described as being 'less drowsy' than the other. What did that really mean? The researchers measured drowsiness on a visual analog scale (VAS). This scale is simply a line that is exactly 10 cm long. Patients are asked to mark somewhere on the line how drowsy they feel with one end of the line representing no drowsiness and the other end representing the maximum possible drowsiness (presumably the maximum drowsiness that you can have and still be awake enough to make a mark on a line). For one drug, the average drowsiness was 3.6 cm at baseline and remained about the same at the end of the study. In the other drug, the average drowsiness declined from 3.6 to 3.3. On the basis of a 3-mm shift, the researchers made the claim of less drowsiness. The 3-mm shift (see Figure 3.3) was indeed statistically significant, but does such a small shift have any practical value?

I was asked to coauthor an editorial discussing this question (Portnoy 2003). We chose a provocative title: 'Is 3-mm Less Drowsiness Important?' It turns out that there is no research on this question. The best information that we could come up with was a study that showed how to establish

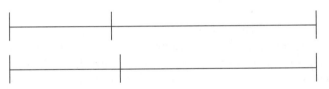

Figure 3.3. A 3mm shift on the 10 cm visual analog scale.

clinical significance for the VAS used in pain measurement (Powell 2001). In that study, children visiting an emergency room were asked to rate their pain on the VAS at 20 minute intervals and also asked to categorize the change from the last time point as either 'heaps better', 'a bit better', 'much the same', 'a bit worse', or 'heaps worse'. The average change in VAS for those patients saying either a bit better or a bit worse was 10 mm.

Once in a while, you will get a researcher to commit to a discussion of this very question. For example, in a study of an educational intervention intended to reduce the number of prescriptions to a drug that is often prescribed inappropriately (Pimlott 2003), researchers found that primary care physicians randomized to an educational intervention did indeed decrease the number of prescriptions to an inappropriate drug (20.3% before and 19.6% after the intervention) while a control group showed an increase (19.8% before to 20.9% after). Although the change was statistically significant ($p = 0.036$), the researchers admit that the size of the change was so small as to be unimportant from a clinical perspective.

3.4.3   How to establish a level of clinical importance

Clinical importance represents a value judgment, and the best way to assess values of your patients is to ask them.

Example: Cancer patients have major problems with fatigue. The only good measure is a self-report, and this can be measured in several different ways:

- Profile of Mood States (POMS), a 65-item scale with a subscale of five items representing fatigue. Each item is rated from 0 to 4.
- Schwartz Cancer Fatigue Scale (SCFS), a 28-item scale with four subscales: physical, emotional, cognitive, and temporal. Each item is rated from 0 to 4.
- General Fatigue Scale (GFS), a 10-item scale with no subscales. Each item is rated from 1 to 10.
- A single question 'what is your level of fatigue today?' with 0 representing 'no fatigue' and 10 representing 'the greatest possible fatigue'.

To establish a minimal level of clinical importance, researchers measured a group of 103 cancer patients before and after initiation of chemotherapy (Schwartz 2002). In addition to getting the four scales, the patients were asked at follow-up whether their fatigue levels had changed and by how much.

If you look at the average change in each scale for those patients who report a small change in fatigue, this represents a minimally important clinical difference. The numbers do not seem to quite match the tables, but the authors suggest that a 5.6 unit shift in POMS, 5.0 for SCFS, 9.7 for GFS, and 2.4 for the single item scale is important. If you divide each of these values by the number of items in the scale, you get values that hover around 1.0 for the first three scales, which is similar to the general recommendation in Guyatt (1998).

Another approach is to get an estimate of the benefits associated with a cure relative to the costs, inconvenience, and other troubles associated with the new treatment. This ratio will provide you with a threshold cure rate that you would demand in order to justify the new treatment. Let us suppose, for example, that the benefits of a cure are five times as valuable as the burden imposed by a new treatment. Since the burdens of the treatment are borne by all who adopt the therapy, but the benefits accrue only to that fraction of patients who are actually cured, you should demand that more than one-fifth of your patients achieve a cure in order for the treatment to achieve a level of clinical importance.

A more sophisticated argument along the same lines appears in Chapter 6, where the ratio of the number needed to treat to the number needed to harm gives you a perspective on how many side effects must be endured in order to achieve one additional cure.

You can also apply an economic argument to establish clinical importance. For example, you can assess the value of a screening program by the proportion of patients discovered with an otherwise undiagnosed disease. When the proportion is high, the overall cost of screening is spread out over a large number of newly diagnosed patients. A screening program has a clinically trivial impact if the proportion of new cases identified is so small that the cost per diagnosis becomes outrageously expensive.

3.4.4 Evaluating negative trials

Establishing a level of clinical importance is especially important for negative trials—trials that fail to achieve statistical significance. You would like some assurance that the trial was negative because a clinically significant change was well outside the range of sampling error. You can look for a confidence interval that is narrow enough to fit entirely inside the range of clinical indifference. You could also look for a justification of the sample size, such as a power calculation.

The problem with a lot of negative trials, though, is that there is too much imprecision in the confidence intervals and no attempt was made before the start of the study to justify the sample size. These negative trials are truly uninformative because you cannot tell if the trial is negative because nothing is going on against having a sample so small that effectively makes it impossible to detect important changes.

How often does this happen? More often than you would like to think. Recall the review of 2,000 schizophrenia trials, where only 3% of the studies had a reasonable sample size.

3.4.5   Evaluating equivalence and non-inferiority trials

Certain studies strive for a 'negative' result. These trials, called equivalence trials, try to demonstrate that a new drug or treatment is comparable to a standard drug or treatment. For example, before the US Food and Drug Administration will approve a generic equivalent for a name brand drug, they require that the generic manufacturer show that the rate and extent of absorption for the generic drug is not much greater (usually not more than 125%) or not much less (usually not less than 80%) than for the name brand drug. This is usually easy to show. In some cases, though, this agency will demand a greater degree of evidence by asking that the generic drug manufacturer show equivalence in the therapeutic benefits of the generic drug.

The goal of an equivalence study is not to show that two drugs are identical, which would be impossible. Instead, you want to show that the difference between the two drugs is no larger than a specified amount.

You should pay extra close attention to the conduct of the research in an equivalence trial. Researchers who are trying to demonstrate that two drugs are equivalent have a built-in incentive to conduct the research haphazardly. The researchers may study patients who were not very sick to begin with, or they may not aggressively work to ensure that patients take their drugs regularly, or they may get a bit sloppy in evaluating the outcome. These problems tend to dilute the differences between the two drugs, making it easier to show that they are equivalent.

There are several approaches that work well when you are trying to show equivalence. The simplest is to compute a confidence interval for the difference between the two groups and see whether it lies entirely inside the range of clinical indifference. Another effective approach is to conduct two tests. If the first test rejects the hypothesis that drug A is inferior by a certain margin to drug B and the second test rejects the hypothesis that drug B is inferior by the same margin to drug A, then you have sufficient evidence of equivalence.

You might be tempted to set up a null hypothesis that the two drugs have the same average effects and when you fail to reject that hypothesis, conclude that the two drugs are equivalent. This approach will not work because you cannot be sure that accepting the null hypothesis was not due to an insufficient sample size.

A similar type of trial, the non-inferiority trial attempts to show that a new drug is not worse by a specified amount from the standard drug (Snapinn 2000). You might be interested in non-inferiority when the new drug is cheaper, more readily tolerated, or has fewer side effects than the standard drug. For such a drug, you would readily adopt it over the standard drug unless you knew that the new drug was much less effective. So you set a non-inferiority margin, and try to assure yourself that the new drug exceeds the non-inferiority margin.

Like the equivalence trial, small details about how the trial was conducted can dilute the differences between two drugs, making it easier to show non-inferiority.

3.5 Counterpoint: Blinding is overrated

There is a strong belief that a study has to be blinded in order to be credible. Some meta-analyses will not include unblinded studies in their summaries in the belief that their quality is too poor (see e.g. Busse 2002; Cooper 2003).

Blinding is just one of many factors that combine to indicate a study's rigor and quality. Although unblinded studies are considered less authoritative than blinded studies, you should not use blinding by itself as a surrogate marker for the quality of the research (Schulz 2002). For example, Rupert Sheldrake conducted a survey of various journals and showed that blinding was used in 85% of all parapsychology research. But it would be a mistake to claim, as Dr. Sheldrake does, that 'Parapsychologists... have been constantly subjected to intense scrutiny by skeptics, and this has made them more rigorous' (http://www.parascope.com/en/articles/blindScience.htm).

There are some situations where blinding is impossible. If one of the treatments in a research study is a bilateral orchiectomy, you cannot blind the study. Sooner or later, your patients are going to notice that something is missing.

Blinding is often achieved through the use of a placebo, but sometimes the price you pay with a placebo is too great to tolerate. In a study of Parkinson's disease (Freed 2002), patients in the treatment group received a transplant of nerve cells injected directly into their brains through two holes drilled into their skulls. The control group received a placebo surgery. Holes were drilled into their skulls also, but no cells were injected. This study was met with a storm of criticism. One of the harsher criticisms (Weijer 2002) had the provocative title, 'I need a placebo like I need a hole in the head.'

In addition, a recent study showed that the benefits of blinding through the use of a placebo effect might be overstated in some contexts (Hrobjartsson 2001). This study compared research studies which had a treatment arm, a placebo arm, and a no-treatment arm. The only difference between the placebo and the no-treatment arm is that the latter is unblinded. These researchers found that with a few exceptions (most notably studies involving pain assessment), there was not a big difference between the placebo arm and the no-treatment arm. So maybe all the fuss about placebos and blinding is overrated. Some of the effects attributed to the placebo are perhaps caused instead by statistical artefacts like regression to the mean or by the tendency of some conditions to resolve spontaneously.

So, is blinding really necessary? It is nice to have, but not at the expense of your ethical principles.

3.6   Summary—Mountain or molehill?

Look carefully at how the researchers measured the outcome in their study.

Did they measure the right thing? You would like to see an outcome of direct interest in your patients.

Did they measure it well? You want an outcome that is valid and reliable and not subject to changes after the start of data collection.

Were the changes clinically important? You want a change that is large enough to have a practical impact in a clinical setting.

3.7   On your own

1.   Review the following abstracts and identify one or more surrogate outcomes. Specify a patient-oriented outcome that might be related to each surrogate outcome.

Effects of disease modifying agents and dietary intervention on insulin resistance and dyslipidemia in inflammatory arthritis: a pilot study. Dessein, P. H., Joffe, B.I., and Stanwix, A.E. *Arthritis Research* 2002, 4:R12 doi:10.1186/ar597. **Abstract:** Patients with rheumatoid arthritis (RA) experience excess cardiovascular disease (CVD). We investigated the effects of disease-modifying antirheumatic drugs (DMARD) and dietary intervention on CVD risk in inflammatory arthritis. Twenty-two patients (17 women; 15 with RA and 7 with spondyloarthropathy) who were insulin resistant ($n = 20$), as determined by the Homeostasis Model Assessment, and/or were dyslipidemic ($n = 11$) were identified. During the third month after initiation of DMARD therapy, body weight, C-reactive protein (CRP), insulin resistance, and lipids were re-evaluated. Results are expressed as median (interquartile range). DMARD therapy together with dietary intervention was associated with weight loss of 4 kg (0–6.5 kg), a decrease in CRP of 14% (6–36%; $p<0.006$), and a reduction in insulin resistance of 36% (26–61%; $p<0.006$). Diet compliers ($n = 15$) experienced decreases of 10% (0–20%) and 3% (0–9%) in total and low-density lipoprotein cholesterol, respectively, as compared with increases of 9% (6–20%; $p < 0.05$) and 3% (0–9%; $p < 0.05$) in diet noncompliers. Patients on methotrexate ($n = 14$) experienced a reduction in CRP of 27 mg/l (6–83 mg/l), as compared with a decrease of 10 mg/l (3.4–13 mg/l; $p = 0.04$) in patients not on methotrexate. Improved cardiovascular risk with DMARD therapy includes a reduction in insulin resistance. Methotrexate use in RA may improve CVD risk through a marked suppression of the acute phase response. Dietary intervention prevented the increase in total and low-density lipoprotein cholesterol upon acute phase response suppression.

This is an open source publication. The full free text is available at: www. arthritis-research.com/4/6/R12

Substituting abacavir for hyperlipidemia-associated protease inhibitors in HAART regimens improves fasting lipid profiles, maintains virologic suppression, and simplifies treatment. Keiser, P.H, Sension, M.G., DeJesus, E., Allan Rodriguez, A., Olliffe, J.F., Williams, V.C., Wakeford, J.H., Snidow, J.W., Shachoy-Clark, A.D., Fleming, J.W., Pakes, G.E. Hernandez, J.E., and for the ESS40003 Study Team. *BMC Infectious Diseases* 2005, 5:2 doi:10.1186/1471–2334–5–2. **Background:** Hyperlipidemia secondary to protease inhibitors (PI) may abate by switching to anti-HIV medications without lipid effects. **Method:** An open-label, randomized pilot study compared changes in fasting lipids and HIV-1 RNA in 104 HIV-infected adults with PI-associated hyperlipidemia (fasting serum total cholesterol >200 mg/dl) who were randomized either to a regimen in which their PI was replaced by abacavir 300 mg twice daily ($n = 52$) or a regimen in which their PI was continued ($n = 52$) for 28 weeks. All patients had undetectable viral loads (HIV-1 RNA <50 copies/ml) at baseline and were naïve to abacavir and non-nucleoside reverse transcriptase inhibitors. **Results:** At baseline, the mean total cholesterol was 243 mg/dl, low density lipoprotein (LDL)-cholesterol 149 mg/dl, high density lipoprotein (HDL)-cholesterol 41 mg/dL, and triglycerides 310 mg/dl. Mean CD4+ cell counts were 551 and 531 cells/mm3 in the abacavir-switch and PI-continuation arms, respectively. At week 28, the abacavir-switch arm had significantly greater least square mean reduction from baseline in total cholesterol (-42 vs. -10 mg/dl, $p < 0.001$), LDL-cholesterol (-14 vs. $+5$ mg/dl, $p = 0.016$), and triglycerides (-134 vs. -36 mg/dl, $p = 0.019$) than the PI-continuation arm, with no differences in HDL-cholesterol ($+0.2$ vs. $+1.3$ mg/dl, $p = 0.583$). A higher proportion of patients in the abacavir-switch arm had decreases in protocol-defined total cholesterol and triglyceride toxicity grades, whereas a smaller proportion had increases in these toxicity grades. At week 28, an intent to treat: missing = failure analysis showed that the abacavir-switch and PI-continuation arms did not differ significantly with respect to proportion of patients maintaining HIV-1 RNA <400 or <50 copies/ml or adjusted mean change from baseline in CD4+ cell count. Two possible abacavir-related hypersensitivity reactions were reported. No significant changes in glucose, insulin, insulin resistance, C-peptide, or waist-to-hip ratios were observed in either treatment arm, nor were differences in these parameters noted between treatments. **Conclusion:** In hyperlipidemic, antiretroviral-experienced patients with HIV-1 RNA levels <50 copies/ml and CD4+ cell counts >500 cells/mm^3, substituting abacavir for hyperlipidemia-associated PIs in combination antiretroviral regimens improves lipid profiles and maintains virologic suppression over a 28-week period, and it simplifies treatment.

This is an open source publication. The full free text is available at: www.biomedcentral.com/1471–2334/5/2.

2. Review the following abstracts and identify the total number of outcome variables. Can you identify one or two outcome measures that should be considered of primary importance?

Effect of reproductive factors on stage, grade and hormone receptor status in early-onset breast cancer. Largent, J.A., Ziogas, A., and Anton-Culver, H. *Breast Cancer Research* 2005, 7:R541-R554 doi:10.1186/bcr1198. **Introduction:** Women younger than 35 years who are diagnosed with breast cancer tend to have more advanced stage tumors and poorer prognoses than do older women. Pregnancy is associated with elevated exposure to estrogen, which may influence the progression of breast cancer in young women. The objective of the present study was to examine the relationship between reproductive events and tumor stage, grade, estrogen receptor, and progesterone receptor status, and survival in women diagnosed with early-onset breast cancer. **Methods:** In a population-based, case–case study of 254 women diagnosed with invasive breast cancer at age under 35 years, odds ratios (ORs) and 95% confidence intervals (CIs) were estimated using unconditional logistic regression with tumor characteristics as dependent variables and adjusting for age and education. Survival analyses also examined the relationship between reproductive events and overall survival. **Results:** Compared with nulliparous women, women with three or more childbirths were more likely to be diagnosed with nonlocalized tumors (OR = 3.1, 95% CI, 1.3–7.7), and early age (<20 years) at first full-term pregnancy was also associated with a diagnosis of breast cancer that was nonlocalized (OR = 3.0, 95% CI, 1.2–7.4) and of higher grade (OR = 3.2, 95% CI, 1.0–9.9). The hazard ratio for death among women with two or more full-term pregnancies, as compared with those with one full-term pregnancy or none, was 2.1 (95% CI, 1.0–4.5), adjusting for stage. Among parous women, those who lactated were at decreased risk for both estrogen receptor and progesterone receptor negative tumors (OR = 0.2, 95% CI, 0.1–0.5, and OR = 0.4, 95% CI, 0.2–0.8, respectively). **Conclusion:** The results of the present study suggest that pregnancy and lactation may influence tumor presentation and survival in women with early-onset breast cancer.

This is an open source publication. The full free text is available at: www.breast-cancer-research.com/content/7/4/R541.

Quality of life, functional outcome, and voice handicap index in partial laryngectomy patients for early glottic cancer. Kandogan, T. and Sanal, A. *BMC Ear, Nose and Throat Disorders* 2005, 5:3 doi:10.1186/1472–6815–5–3. **Background:** In this study, we aim to gather information about the quality of life issues, functional outcomes and voice problems facing early glottic cancer patients treated with the surgical techniques such as laryngofissure cordectomy, fronto-lateral laryngectomy, or cricohyoidopexi. In particular, consistency of life and voice quality issues with the laryngeal tissue excised during surgery is examined. In addition, the effects of aryte-noidectomy to the life and voice quality are also studied. **Methods:** Twenty-nine male patients were enrolled voluntarily in the study. The average age was 53.9 years. Three out of ten patients with laryngofissure cordectomy also had arytenoidectomy. Eleven patients had fronto-lateral laryngectomy with Tucker reconstruction, two of which also had arytenoidectomy. There were eight patients with cricohyoidopexi and bilateral functional neck dissection. Three of these patients also had arytenoidectomy. In bilateral functional neck dissection cases, spinal accessory nerve was preserved and level V of the neck was not dissected. None of the patients had neither radiotherapy nor voice therapy. Cordectomy patients never had a temporary tracheotomy or were connected to a feeding tube. Data was collected for 13 months for the cordectomy group, 14 months for fronto-lateral laryngectomy and cricohyoidopexi groups on average post-operatively. Statistical analysis in this study was carried out using the one-way analysis of variance, and the *Post hoc* group comparisons were made after Bonferroni and Scheffé procedures. In order to determine the effects of arytenoidectomy, a regression analysis is carried out to see if there are statistical differences in answers given to the survey questions among patients who were arytenoidectomized during their surgeries. **Results:** There was a statistically significant difference between cordectomy and cricohyoidopexi group in answers to the University of Washington–Quality of Life–Revised survey part 1. ($p = 0$). A statistically significant difference was also established between cordectomy and fronto-lateral laryngectomy groups, as well as between cordectomy and cricohyoidopexi groups in answers to the University of Washington–Quality of Life–Revised survey part 2. ($p = 0.036$ and $p = 0.009$, respectively). Cricohyoidopexi group has given the lowest scores and the cordectomy group has given the highest scores in three survey questions representing the quality of life, performances and new voices. These ranges are also consistent with the laryngeal tissue excised during surgery (cricohyoidopexi > fronto-lateral laryngectomy > cordectomy). There was no statistically significant difference between groups in Performance Status Scale for Head and Neck cancer patients instrument. The difference between the Voice Handicap Index and Voice Handicap Index (functional); Voice Handicap Index (physical) and Voice Handicap Index (emotional) scores in three patient groups was not significant either. All of the patients evaluated that their new voices have similar functional, physical and emotional impact on their life. Decanulation and oral feeding times of cricohyoidopexi and fronto-lateral laryngectomy patients are found to be significantly longer than cordectomy patients. Lastly, the removal of arytenoid does not have any significant adverse effects on the quality of life, the functional outcomes, or the quality of voice. **Conclusion:** In the present study, all patients with early glottic cancer, treated with different surgical techniques reported fairly good quality of life outcomes, functional results and voice qualities. This study also finds that the removal of arytenoid does not have any adverse effects on the quality of life and voice from the patients' point of view.

This is an open source publication. The full free text is available at www.biomedcentral.com/1472–6815/5/3.

3.   Review the following abstracts. These reports represent studies where no blinding was done. How critical is the lack of blinding in these studies? What attempts at partial blinding could have been attempted?

Measurement of tracheal temperature is not a reliable index of total respiratory heat loss in mechanically ventilated patients. *Critical Care* 2001, 5:24–30 doi:10.1186/cc974. **Background:** Minimizing total respiratory heat loss is an important goal during mechanical ventilation. The aim of the present study was to evaluate whether changes in tracheal temperature (a clinical parameter that is easy to measure) are reliable indices of total respiratory heat loss in mechanically ventilated patients. **Method:** Total respiratory heat loss was measured, with three different methods of inspired gas conditioning, in ten sedated patients. The study was randomized and of a crossover design. Each patient was ventilated for three consecutive 24-h periods with a heated humidifier (HH), a hydrophobic heat-moisture exchanger (HME) and a hygroscopic HME. Total respiratory heat loss and tracheal temperature were simultaneously obtained in each patient. Measurements were obtained during each 24-h study period after 45 min, and 6 and 24 h. **Results:** Total respiratory heat loss varied from 51 to 52 cal/min with the HH, from 100 to 108 cal/min with the hydrophobic HME, and from 92 to 102 cal/min with the hygroscopic HME ($p < 0.01$). Simultaneous measurements of maximal tracheal temperatures revealed no significant differences between the HH (35.7–35.9°C) and either HME (hydrophobic 35.3–35.4°C, hygroscopic 36.2–36.3°C). **Conclusion:** In intensive care unit (ICU) mechanically ventilated patients, total respiratory heat loss was twice as much with either hydrophobic or hydroscopic HME than with the HH. This suggests that a much greater amount of heat was extracted from the respiratory tract by the HMEs than by the HH. Tracheal temperature, although simple to measure in ICU patients, does not appear to be a reliable estimate of total respiratory heat loss.

This is an open source publication. The full free text is available at wwwccforum.com/content/5/1/024.

Re-examining age, race, site, and thermometer type as variables affecting temperature measurement in adults—a comparison study. Smith, L.S. *BMC Nursing* 2003, 2:1 doi:10.1186/1472–6955–2–1. **Background:** As a result of the recent international vigilance regarding disease assessment, accurate measurement of body temperature has become increasingly important. Yet, trusted low-tech, portable mercury glass thermometers are no longer available. Thus, comparing accuracy of mercury-free thermometers with mercury devices is essential. Study purposes were (1) to examine age, race, site as variables affecting temperature measurement in adults, and (2) to compare clinical accuracy of low-tech Galinstan-in-glass device to mercury-in-glass at oral, axillary, groin, and rectal sites in adults. **Methods:** Setting 176 bed accredited health care facility, rural northwest US Participants Convenience sample ($n = 120$) of hospitalized persons = 18 years old. Instruments Temperatures (°F) measured at oral, skin (simultaneous), immediately followed by rectal sites with four each mercury-glass (BD) and Galinstan-glass (Geratherm) thermometers; 10 minute dwell times. **Results:** Participants averaged 61.6 years (SD 17.9), 188 pounds (SD 55.3); 61% female; race: 85% White, 8.3% Native Am., 4.2% Hispanic, 1.7 % Asian, 0.8% Black. For both mercury and Galinstan-glass thermometers, within-subject temperature readings were highest rectally; followed by oral, then skin sites. Galinstan assessments demonstrated rectal sites 0.91°F > oral and 1.3°F > skin sites. Devices strongly correlated between and across sites. Site difference scores between devices showed greatest variability at skin sites; least at rectal site. 95% confidence intervals of difference scores by site (°F): oral ($0.142 - 0.265$), axilla ($0.167 - 0.339$), groin ($0.037 - 0.321$), and rectal ($-0.111 - 0.111$). Race correlated with age, temperature readings each site and device. **Conclusion:** Temperature readings varied by age, race. Mercury readings correlated with Galinstan thermometer readings at all sites. Site mean differences between devices were considered clinically insignificant. Still considered the gold standard, mercury-glass thermometers may no longer be available worldwide. Therefore, mercury-free, environmentally safe low-tech Galinstan-in-glass may be an appropriate replacement. This is especially important as we face new, internationally transmitted diseases.

This is an open source publication. The full free text is available at www.biomedcentral.com/1472–6955/2/1.

4 What Do the Other Witnesses Say? Corroborating Evidence

4.1 Introduction

In a criminal trial, the prosecutor will sometimes try to demonstrate that the defendant had:

- the means to commit the crime;
- the motive to commit the crime; and
- the opportunity to commit the crime.

All three elements are not really necessary for a conviction—many people are convicted without the need to show a motive, for example. But when the prosecution can identify a motive, that makes their case that much more convincing.

This analogy also holds for research studies. Some studies are so well done that their evidence alone would be enough to convince you. Other studies, however, provide only weak evidence. But when this evidence is combined with other information, the evidence can become quite strong.

Sir Austin Bradford Hill outlined a series of tests that you could use to evaluate whether an association between an environmental factor and disease was credible (Hill 1965). These criteria are not perfect. A strong criticism of Hill's criteria appears in a classic textbook on epidemiology by Kenneth Rothman and Sander Greenland (Rothmann 1998). Rothman and Greenland point out that none of Hill's criteria (with the exception of temporality) are necessary or sufficient for establishing causation.

While their criticisms are important to remember, I believe they missed the point of Hill's original article. No one criterion by itself will establish the credibility of a research study if it is present and no one criterion will destroy the credibility of a study if it is absent. You should look at the aggregate impact of these factors. When most of them are present, they add to the credibility of a study. When most of them are absent, they weaken the credibility of the study. As Sir Hill himself notes:

> All scientific work is incomplete—whether it be observational or experimental. All scientific work is liable to be upset or modified by advancing knowledge. This does not confer upon us a freedom to ignore

the knowledge we already have, or to postpone the action that it appears to demand at a given time. Who knows, asked Robert Browning, but that the world may end tonight? True, but on available evidence, most of us make ready to commute on the 8:30 next day. (Hill 1965)

4.1.1   Case study: A drug treatment that only works in black patients

There has been a lot of published research that shows that heart disease is different and more deadly among black patients. Some possible explanations of these differences involve the renin-angiotensin system in bioavailability of nitric oxide. In a study that seemed to show no overall differences in efficacy for a drug treatment (hydralazine plus isosorbide dinitrate), for treating congestive heart failure, there was nevertheless the suggestion that this treatment might be effective when analysis was restricted to just the black patients in the study. This study, however, was not designed to look for race-specific effects, so the results had to be treated as preliminary. The authors of one review stated that 'prospective trials involving large numbers of black patients are needed to further clarify their response to therapy' (Carson 1999). With this justification, a new randomized trial, recruiting just black patients, was begun. This study did indeed show that the two drugs were effective among these black patients (Taylor 2004), and became one of the first examples of a therapy recommended solely for a specific racial subgroup.

The concept of using race or ethnicity in medical decisions is controversial, because of the potential for misuse and abuse of this information (Bhopal 1997). There is also debate about whether there are enough genetic variations among different racial and ethnic groups to justify treating them as distinct groups. The authors of the second study skirted this issue by using the phrase 'patients who self-identify as black'.

The important lesson, though, is that no study should be examined in isolation. You should always be looking for corroborating evidence. The subgroup finding (Carson 1999) was indeed a weak form of evidence, but it was supported by several mechanistic explanations described above. When these results were replicated in an independent study, the evidence in favor of this controversial treatment became overwhelmingly persuasive.

4.1.2   What do the other witnesses say? What to look for

Additional details, both within and outside the research study can provide support for an otherwise weak form of evidence.

Is there a strong association? A treatment that has a large impact is unlikely to become undone by small flaws in the research.

Is there a dose-response pattern? A treatment that shows stronger effects when given in stronger doses adds credibility to a study because it reduces the credibility of certain biasing factors.

Is the association consistent? A result that is replicated across diverse populations using diverse research designs adds credibility because it is unlikely that a particular flaw in the research could affect all these studies in the same way.

Is the association specific? A treatment that cures 'everything' lacks specificity. You should mistrust such a treatment because it is likely to be caused by a global bias in the health of the treated and untreated patients. In contrast, a treatment that cures one particular condition, but not others would rule out such a global bias.

Is the association biologically plausible? A treatment that has no sound biological basis has to pass a higher threshold of evidence than a treatment that has a plausible biological mechanism.

Is there a conflict of interest? Research that is untainted by commercial temptations is more credible because the researchers have no financial incentive to skew the research results.

Is there any evidence of fraud? Research that is carefully reviewed reduces the chances of deliberate falsification of the data.

4.2   Is there a strong association?

No research is perfect, and there is always the possibility that some unaccounted for factor might have caused the results seen in the research rather than the treatment being studied. This is less likely to be the case, however, when there is a strong association—in other words, when the treatment has a large effect on the outcome. By contrast, a weak association—one where the treatment only has a small effect on the outcome—is less persuasive because any small bias or problem with the research could swamp the result.

Example: In a retrospective chart review of surgical treatment of peripheral vascular disease (Logar 2005), patients received either surgical revascularization or amputation. The risk of gangrene was substantially higher in the amputation group (odds ratio =19, 95% CI 14–26). Even though this was not a randomized study and the results were assessed retrospectively, the very large difference between the two groups still makes the results persuasive.

Perhaps the best example of a strong association is the link between cigarette smoking and lung cancer. The studies that established this link in the 1950s and 1960s were not perfect. They did not use randomization, because it would be unethical. They often relied on retrospective data, because of the long latency period between exposure and the development of cancer. They did not have a perfect control group for many of these studies, and there were a lot of potential confounding variables that had to be accounted for. Nevertheless, these studies showed a large effect, typically a tenfold or greater risk of lung cancer when smokers were compared to nonsmokers. So while these studies did have numerous flaws and biases, it would be very difficult to find something that, independent of cigarette smoking, had a tenfold or greater effect on lung cancer. It would take a bias or flaw that severe to produce such a lopsided finding.

What is a strong association/large effect? There is no magic number. A commonly quoted rule of thumb is that an odds ratio or relative risk of two or greater represents a large effect. Any treatment that can double the chances of a cure or cut the risk of side effects in half is considered a strong association that is unlikely to be due to small biases in the research. Ratios less than two are less credible because they could more readily be caused by small biases or flaws in the research.

The problem with this rule of thumb is when it is taken too literally. Rothman (1998) points out correctly that 'a strong association serves only to rule out hypotheses that the association is entirely due to one weak unmeasured confounder or other source of experimenter bias.' It is a mistake to blindly trust any odds ratio greater than two. Some research studies have major flaws that could artefactually produce odds ratios of two or larger. It is also a mistake to totally disregard any odds ratio less than two. Some research studies are so well conducted that even a small odds ratio is credible.

4.3   Is there a dose-response pattern?

If a treatment or exposure is given in varying doses, and increasing doses lead to increasing effects on the outcome, then you have a dose-response pattern. Having such a pattern generally adds to the credibility of the study. The reason for this is that many (but not all) biases and flaws in a research study would affect all doses of a treatment equally, and it is only a few flaws and biases that would produce an artefactual dose-response pattern. For example, if a drug is effective only because the control subjects were poorly chosen, then the difference in the outcome should be the same for all levels of the treatment. This sort of bias could not produce a dose-response pattern and could not serve as a credible alternative.

Example: In a study of respiratory health (Maziak 2005), the degree of environmental tobacco smoke (ETS) was cumulated across multiple self-reports indices to create a composite score where a low value represents a minimal exposure to ETS and high value represents a large exposure to ETS. This composite score showed a strong dose-response pattern for several symptoms of respiratory distress, making for stronger evidence that ETS has adverse effects on health than a simple comparison of all patients exposed to some level of ETS compared to patients with no exposure to ETS.

Some biases and flaws, though, could still produce a dose-response pattern. Suppose you are looking at groups of patients who have good, better, and best levels of exercise. There may be a third factor, such as nutrition, where those patients in the good exercise group typically have good nutrition, but those in the best exercise group have typically the best nutrition. Then this nutrition factor might produce a dose-response pattern of bias which the naive researcher might mistake for an effect of exercise itself.

Furthermore, not all treatments can or should be expected to produce a dose-response pattern. Sometimes medicines have a threshold effect; any dose below a certain point is completely ineffective, and any dose above that point produces a roughly comparable effect. Similarly, some exposures are perfectly safe up to a certain point, but beyond that point they are uniformly fatal. The best example, though the final word has not been written yet, is in the consumption of wine. The evidence to date suggests that people who consume a small amount of wine daily have a lower risk of heart attacks and therefore a better overall mortality profile than those who consume no wine or those who consume a lot of wine.

Rothman (1998) is also critical of this criteria and points out that birth order shows a dose-response relationship with Down's syndrome with first born children being less likely to have this condition. This relationship however is just a reflection of the fact that age of the parents is positively associated with Down's syndrome. Older parents are more likely to have children with Down's syndrome, and birth order and age of the parents shows a strong negative correlation.

4.4   Is the association consistent?

The most common request in research is: 'I won't believe it until I see it replicated.' It is one of the first things that I would look for if the evidence in a particular study is weak. The link between cigarette smoking and lung cancer provides the best example of the value of replication. As noted above, any single study of smoking had potential flaws. So when the first study appeared, skeptics could produce a reason (call it A) that might explain away the results of the study. A second and different study would appear, and skeptics could find a different reason (call it B) that might explain away the results of that study as well. And for the third study, they offered up C and for the fourth study, they offered up D. Eventually, though, these series of claims, A, B, C, D, . . . became less credible than the hypothesis that smoking causes cancer because those series of counter-arguments also needed to be skeptically evaluated. It was the strength of a wide range of studies, not any single study, that produced convincing evidence of a link between lung cancer and smoking.

You have to be careful to look at the type of replication. Mindless replication that just repeats the same experiment over and over again will just end up producing the exact same biases. In the real world, different researchers try different approaches. Although there is not always an explicit plan, a series of replications will often be varied enough so that a confounding factor that might be present in one study is unlikely to be present in all studies.

In fact, researchers often do have an explicit plan to replicate in such a way that any biasing factor in one study will be eliminated in another study (Rosenbaum 2001). This reference has some fascinating examples and the best one is from Economics rather than Medicine.

There is a huge debate among economists about the impact of minimum-wage laws. Liberal economists will argue that minimum-wage laws help ensure that low-paid workers get enough wages to stay above the poverty level. Conservative economists will argue that these laws increase unemployment because they push wages beyond the value that some unskilled workers might offer to a company.

One way to test this is to see what happens to the employment rate when the minimum wage increases. New Jersey has a higher minimum wage than its neighboring states, so you could look at what happens to the employment in New Jersey each time they increase the minimum wage. It turns out that when New Jersey increased its minimum wage, the employment rate did not change relative to the rate in a neighboring state (Pennsylvania).

You could argue quite validly that this is a weak form of evidence. You are comparing New Jersey apples to Pennsylvania oranges. If you tried to strengthen this evidence by looking at other times when New Jersey's minimum wage jumped, it would not be at all convincing because you would be making the same apples-to-oranges comparison. It turns out, though, that there was a different sort of replication. When the US government raised the minimum wage, it raised the minimum wage in Pennsylvania, but not in New Jersey which already had its minimum wage set at the level that the federal government had proposed.

Interestingly, there was no change in the unemployment rate in Pennsylvania relative to New Jersey. Again this is a weak form of evidence because you are comparing Pennsylvania apples to New Jersey oranges. But the two studies combined are quite strong. Both comparisons would almost certainly be flawed, but they would almost have to be flawed in opposite directions. When a result is consistent across studies that should be biased in opposite directions, you can be confident that the true result is stronger than any bias in the research.

4.5   Is the association specific?

A new therapy that makes narrow claims about the outcomes that it can influence provides greater credibility for a research study. In contrast, a new therapy that seems to influence a wide range of health outcomes is less persuasive. Something that cures everything should make you suspicious that perhaps the groups being compared are not apples and apples. It may mean instead that the research design ended up implicitly selecting healthier patients in the treatment group and sicker patients in the control group. In contrast, an association that is specific to a particular disease or condition to the exclusion of other diseases or conditions has greater credibility. It is harder to find a research flaw that would affect the association with one disease and not with other diseases.

Example: In a cross-sectional study from a national representative sample of 3,032 people aged 25–74 (Goodwin 2002), researchers assessed the presence of self-reported respiratory and lung disease and various measures of mental health. Panic attacks were related to respiratory disease after adjusting for demographics and co-morbid disorders, but other conditions, such as depression, anxiety, and alcohol/substance abuse were not. The evidence in a cross-sectional study like this with self-reported outcomes would normally be weak, but the fact that the effects of lung disease were specific to panic attacks added some strength to this finding. The authors also note that this work replicated previous findings of a relationship between lung disease and panic attacks, but also admit that there is no known mechanism to explain this association.

A good example of a therapy that makes overly broad and nonspecific claims is craniosacral therapy. This is an alternative medicine practice that involves

> deeply listening to the fluctuations of the cerebrospinal fluid within the Craniosacral system. The fluctuation of the cerebrospinal fluid creates a variety of tides with in the system. As the practitioner—from a place of stillness—listens to these internal tides, the client's system begins to access its own inner resources . . . perhaps a little like finding keys to previously locked doors. The cerebrospinal fluid—as it bathes and protects the brain and spinal cord—carries an intelligence and potency, which becomes mixed with other bodily fluids via the dural membranes. Craniosacral therapists learn to listen deeply to the system, tapping into its inherent intelligence, focusing on the system remembering its original blueprint of health. The therapist encourages the client's system to access its resources, offering new choices and possibilities for the system at every level. Training, then, includes deep perceptual and centering skills as well as extensive study of the anatomy, physiology, and inherent motion of the craniosacral system. (www.craniosacraltherapy.org/FAQ.htm)

Practitioners of craniosacral therapy offer a wide and nonspecific array of conditions of symptoms that it claims to help.

> Impingement of cranial nerves or spinal nerves, left-right imbalances, head injuries, confusion, feelings of compression or pressure, anxiety, depression, circulatory disorders, organ dysfunctions, learning difficulties, neuro-endocrine problems, TMJ and dental problems, and trauma of all kinds—birth, falls, accidents and other injuries, physical, sexual or emotional abuse, PTSD, loss/grief, surgery, anesthesia—all are good indicators that a visit to your craniosacral therapist will be helpful. (www.craniosacraltherapy.org/FAQ.htm)

> Some conditions that commonly respond well to treatment include: Autism, Central nervous system disorders, Chronic back pain, Migraine headaches, Neurovascular disorders, Immune disorders, Post-traumatic stress disorder, Fibromyalgia, and Learning disabilities. (www.fitnessandmassage.com/CST.html)

An exposure that affects a single disease provides more credible evidence than an exposure that affects a broad range of diseases. Applying this to claims about therapy, the conclusion would be that *a therapy that claims to cure everything probably cures nothing*. Stated less extremely, you should use greater caution and demand a greater level of evidence for any therapy that makes overly broad claims of efficacy.

Specificity is so important because many flaws in research, such as poor choice of the control group or failure to adequately blind the treatment, will tend to exaggerate the effectiveness of a therapy across all disease conditions. It puts a pair of rose-colored glasses on the researchers' eyes.

You can make a similar statement about exposures. Many flaws in a study examining the harmful effects of an exposure will show that exposure to be harmful across a broad array of effects.

Effects that are very specific are more credible because it is harder to find a flaw that would cause a treatment to be effective for one disease but not other diseases. It is harder to find a flaw that would cause an exposure to be harmful in only one specific area.

A savvy researcher can exploit specificity to strengthen the credibility of their findings. Suppose an epidemiologist is examining the effects of a toxic exposure, such as carbon monoxide. You cannot randomly assign patients in such a study because of ethical constraints, so instead you choose an observational study where one of the groups is exposed by the nature of their job to excessive amounts of carbon monoxide, such as toll booth operators.

When the epidemiologist compares these workers to a control group, they would normally ask about symptoms such as shortness of breath, dizziness, nausea, and headaches which are associated with carbon monoxide exposure. But they will often also ask about symptoms that are unrelated to this exposure, such as watery eyes, itchy skin, and sneezing.

If the exposed group rated all the symptoms higher than the controls, then you would know that toll booth workers just like to complain more about problems in general. But when they report higher levels only for those symptoms specific to carbon monoxide poisoning, you have greater confidence because you have eliminated a possible alternate explanation for these findings.

Specificity is, by itself, not a perfect indicator of causality. Certain exposures, such as cigarette smoking cause a very broad and nonspecific set of diseases. Certain drugs, such as aspirin, are effective for a wide range of illnesses.

You should not discount the possible benefits of a therapy just because it is nonspecific. Just be cautious. The broader the claims, the more caution you should use.

4.6 Is the association biologically plausible?

'Extraordinary claims require extraordinary proof.' This is the mantra of skeptical thinkers and has been proven useful for evaluating claims that fall outside the mainstream of science. This is part of the network of corroborating evidence that we demand as we review research claims in medical journal articles as well.

You should consider a claim to be extraordinary if there is no plausible mechanism that would explain how the therapy works. You should not automatically reject belief in therapies without a biological mechanism, but you should subject these beliefs to a higher standard of proof. In contrast, the presence of a plausible mechanism can strengthen an otherwise weak conclusion.

Example: In a study of premature births in an agricultural community (Eskenazi 2004), researchers measured metabolite levels of various pesticides in the blood of pregnant Latino women. They then documented the length of the women's pregnancies and the birth weight and size of the newborn infant. Certain pesticides were associated with a decrease in the pregnancy length, and the authors cite the ability of these pesticides to stimulate contraction of the uterus. This mechanism strengths the evidence for relationship between pesticide exposure and premature delivery.

Example: In a study of risk factors for Alzheimer's disease (Tyas 2001), a cohort of older patients was surveyed for a variety of factors and then followed for five years to see who would develop Alzheimer's disease. Patients with occupational exposure to fumigants or defoliants had an increased risk of developing Alzheimer's. Exposure to excessive noise appeared to decrease the risk of Alzheimer's. To evaluate each of these claims, the authors discussed whether a plausible biological mechanism existed. Fumigants and defoliants have well documented neurological effects, which makes the association with Alzhiemer's disease more plausible. There was no plausible mechanism to explain how excessive noise could reduce the risk of Alzheimer's so the authors suggested that this finding was probably just a fluke.

Example: In a systematic overview of research on cervical neoplasia (Mandelblatt 1999), the researchers noted an interaction between the presence of human papilloma virus and HIV. The data suggest that the association between HPV and cervical neoplasia is stronger among women who are HIV-positive. The authors suggest several possible mechanisms to explain this interaction:

> Biological mechanisms through which cellular immunosuppression could facilitate the oncogenic effects of HPV include prolonging the length of time of an HPV infection, increasing HPV viral load, allowing for more rapid HPV replication, persistence, or progression, or impacting on Langerhans' cells. Enhanced oncogenicity of HPV in HIV-infected women is also supported by clinical observations of more rapidly progressive disease and higher rates of recurrence among HIV-positive compared with HIV-negative women with HPV. Indirect evidence also links cellular immune responses and HPV. For example, there are increases in both HPV and CN in transplant patients, pregnant women, aged women, and women with AIDS. Cellular immune suppression also seems to increase the risk of anal neoplasia among HIV-positive men with anal HPV infection, where risk of neoplasia increases with increasing level of immunosuppression. Preliminary data also suggest a molecular interaction between HIV and HPV, where the HIV-1 tat protein transactivates HPV and effects expression of HPV-E2 and the E6 and E7 oncoproteins.

Example: In a review of the research showing reduction of disease risk among people who consume lots of fruits and vegetables (Lampe 1999), the authors suggest several reasons why fruits and vegetables might have a protective effect 'including modulation of detoxification enzymes, stimulation of the immune system, reduction of platelet aggregation, modulation of cholesterol synthesis and hormone metabolism, reduction of blood pressure, and antioxidant, antibacterial, and antiviral effects.' The authors admit, though, that some of these mechanisms are not well established because they have been derived only in animal models and in petri dishes.

Actually, animal research has come under a lot of criticism recently, because of the limited ability to extrapolate results of other species to man. But this research has great value when it helps establish a mechanism for understanding how a new medicine might work. It then becomes a piece of corroborating evidence to support the research done directly on humans.

4.7   Is there a conflict of interest?

Sir Austin Bradford Hill did not mention commercial biases back in 1965, but these have, sad to say, become an important consideration in evaluating today's research.

When a potential conflict of interest is brought to your attention, you need to approach the research cautiously, and you should rightly demand extra evidence. Do not turn into a statistical nihilist, though, and disregard any research with a potential conflict of interest.

Do commercial ties influence research findings? There are many documented cases where money does alter the research. Perhaps the best understood conflict of interest involves the tobacco companies. Financial support from tobacco companies has a large and quantifiable impact on the findings of a study. Articles on passive smoking written by authors affiliated with the tobacco industry were far more likely to conclude that passive smoking was not harmful (Barnes 1998). A review of studies on the economic effects of laws restricting smoking (Scollo 2003) showed that tobacco affiliations were associated with greater use of subjective outcomes, a lower rate of peer review, and a greater tendency to report negative economic impacts.

Support or commercial ties with pharmaceutical companies can also be troublesome. At least thirty studies have examined whether authors with commercial ties come up with more favorable conclusions about the drugs they are studying. A review of these studies, (Lexchin 2003) showed that studies were four times more likely to reach conclusions favorable to the company's product when the researchers were supported by the drug company. The authors offered five possible explanations:

1. Drug companies might preferentially support and test only those drugs that have especially good prospects.
2. The drug company sponsored trials could be of poorer quality and therefore more likely to draw contradictory conclusions.
3. Researchers might deliberately chose the 'wrong' dose of the standard drug offered in the control group, leading to a higher rate of efficacy for the new drug, fewer side effects noted for the new drug, or both.
4. Drug companies might preferentially publish only the studies that support the use of the new drug.
5. Drug companies might deliberately target symposiums, since the lack of peer review might allow them to make stronger statements about their drugs than the data itself would support.

Another problem is that authors rarely disclose possible conflicts. A review of disclosure of conflicts of interest (Hussain 2001) calculated the rate of disclosure at 1.4% (52 out of 3,642), a number that is far too low to be credible. If authors fail to report potential conflicts of interest, it may be out of the stubborn belief that commercial ties only influence *other* people (Boyd 2003).

Charges of financial conflict of interest are sometimes a 'red herring' that is intended to distract from a discussion of the merits of the research. Stephen Senn tells an interesting story about himself (Senn 2001) where such a charge was leveled. Senn is a famous statistician with over 190 publications. Because of his stellar reputation, he is widely sought out as a statistical consultant to the pharmaceutical industry. In a discussion with an academic researcher, though, Senn was informed that his 'source of employment' meant that his recommendations about the proper analysis of crossover trials were worthless. It did not matter that Senn had written the definitive textbook on that very subject (Senn 1993).

So how should you approach a research article where the authors have declared a conflict of interest? You should be cautious, but not cynical. If the research is objective, well documented, and subject to external review, then you should not let financial conflict of interest exert a veto power over the findings. On the other hand, an editorial article or opinion piece written by an author with commercial ties to a product being discussed in the editorial is very troublesome (Angel 1996).

Is there an explicit assurance from the author that the industry support still allowed the author to independently assess the data and to publish the results without first getting approval from the sponsor? A reasonable review period by the sponsor is acceptable as long the final decision to publish rests with the author and not the sponsor. A 2001 revision to the statement on publication ethics from the International Committee of Medical Journal Editors (Davidoff 2001) highlights how important this assurance is.

4.8   Is there any evidence of fraud?

Another consideration not covered by Sir Austin Bradford Hill is fraud. This is also another sad development in research that you need to be concerned about. Research fraud is

> the intentional fabrication or falsification of data or results, plagiarism, or other similarly deceptive practices that seriously deviate from those that are commonly accepted within the scientific community for proposing (e.g., in grant proposals), conducting, or reporting research. It does not include honest error or honest differences in interpretations or judgments of data. (www.jhsph.edu/ora/fraud.html)

It is almost impossible for the average reader to detect fraud in a journal publication.

Journals can protect against fraudulent (and inadvertent) changes in the research protocol by insisting that researchers present the original research protocol to the peer reviewers along with the paper itself (Hawkey 2001). The peer reviewers could then look for any deviations from the original plan that might indicate an attempt to deceive or mislead the readers.

Sometimes a careful review of the numbers in a study can highlight the possibility of fraud. If a study used randomization, for example, watch out if there is an unexpected and unexplained deviation from a 50–50 split between treatment and control. Replication of research findings is also a good protection against fraud. Finally, you have to rely on people who have inside knowledge to come forward when they see evidence of fraud.

Example: In 2001, the *Journal of the American Medical Association* (*JAMA*) published a study of celecoxib (Silverstein 2000). It showed that celecoxib had fewer side effects than competing drugs. The rates of stomach and intestinal ulcers after six months were far lower than the rates of two competing drugs. M. Michael Wolfe wrote a strongly supportive editorial in that same issue of *JAMA* (Lichtenstein 2000). Later, Wolfe discovered the same study as reported to the US Food and Drug Administration (FDA). The drug company's report to the FDA showed that the original plan for the study was to study side effects for a full year. Almost all of the side effects found during the second six months were in patients taking celecoxib, and when you combined the second six months of data with the first, most of the advantages for celecoxib disappeared. The authors of the *JAMA* study argued that the high dropout rate in the second half of the study made the rates based on a full year of data unreliable, but even if this were so, the authors still had an obligation to present the full year's data to allow readers to make up their own mind.

4.9 Counterpoint: Biological plausibility is overrated

An absolute demand for biological plausibility fails to acknowledge that many successful medical interventions were adopted before a mechanism was discovered that explained how and why that intervention worked. Gregor Mendel developed an extensive set of rules on inheritance. This theory was perfectly valid at the time it was developed, even though it took another century before Watson and Crick developed the structure of DNA as the mechanism to support Mendel's rules on inheritance.

Sometimes the problem with biological plausibility is that there is too much of it rather than too little. In some situations, you can find sound biological explanations for diametrically opposite conclusions. Trying to find out what the truth is in this situation is like navigating a minefield. Here's a comment on the various mechanistic explanations on why COX-2 inhibitors might increase the risk of heart disease (Kimmel 2005):

Nonaspirin nonsteroidal anti-inflammatory drugs (NSAIDs) include those that inhibit both the cyclooxygenase-1 (COX-1) isoenzyme and the COX-2 isoenzyme (nonselective NSAIDs) and those that are more selective for the COX-2 isoenzyme (COX-2 selective inhibitors, herein called COX-2 inhibitors). Nonselective NSAIDs may reduce the risk for myocardial infarction (MI) by inhibiting platelet aggregation (1–3). On the other hand, studies have postulated that COX-2 inhibitors increase the risk for atherothrombotic events because they inhibit prostacyclin, which may increase thrombotic tendencies and vascular injury without the beneficial effect of platelet inhibition derived from COX-1 inhibition (4). However, COX-2 inhibitors may also reduce cardiovascular risk by inhibiting vascular inflammation, improving endothelial dysfunction, and enhancing coronary plaque stability (5–8). These effects may differ among COX-2 inhibitors. Along with potential differences in blood pressure effects (9), recent evidence suggests that celecoxib and rofecoxib may differ in their effects on endothelial dysfunction and oxidative stress (8).

This is difficult to read, but as I understand it, there is a plausible mechanism for just about any finding that you can think of with respect to COX-2 inhibitors and heart disease.

It is also difficult to get consensus on what is plausible. For example, several studies have demonstrated that a randomly selected group of patients who received prayer had better health outcomes than patients in a control group. Is there a plausible explanation for this? An atheist/agnostic would come up with a different answer than a religious person would.

Another problem is that some researchers see biological plausibility as a license to manufacture an obscure scientific framework for a result that otherwise could not be supported. For example, an article in the 2001 Christmas holiday issue of the *British Medical Journal* (Leibovici 2001) studied the effects of remote intercessory retrospective prayer. This researcher collected medical records of patients with severe blood infections. These were retrospective records, and the patients were hospitalized anywhere from four to ten years earlier. These records were randomly divided into two groups and then one group of records was prayed for. Then the charts were reviewed. Although there was no difference in mortality, the length of stay and duration of fever were reduced by a statistically significant amount ($p=0.01$ and 0.04 respectively).

This study was intended, I suspect, not to be taken seriously, but instead to highlight some of the general methodological problems with research into the effects of prayer. But another article in the same journal (Olshansky 2003) took the study quite seriously and tried to develop a plausible mechanism to explain how an intervention could affect events that occurred four to ten years earlier.

Models of space and time permitting bi-directional interactions between present and past exist. A current image of the topology of the space-time continuum includes wormholes that link remote regions, when space-time is pinched or folded. Some physicists hypothesise that Calabi-Yau space might allow bi-directional interactions between past and future. These possibilities cannot be dismissed.

This is an example of a search for a plausible mechanism that ignores other choices which are far simpler. The first explanation is that this was just an unfortunate division of the medical charts. After all, the tests in this study were performed at an alpha level of 0.05, which means there is a small but real chance that this finding is just a false positive result. A second explanation is fraud. I would be very hesitant to accuse anyone of fraud, but I would still embrace that possibility before I embraced the possibility that a pinch or fold in space-time occurred right between the two piles of medical records.

Another example of how supporters will stretch an obscure theory to fit their beliefs is discussed in a critical review of some of the mechanistic claims of homeopathy (Park 1997). This paper remarks that proponents of homeopathic medicine have invoked chaos theory on their behalf. One of the central tenets of chaos theory is that small changes in the initial state of a nonlinear system can lead to large changes further on in time. The analogy that is commonly used is that the flapping of a butterfly's wings in China today could cause a hurricane in Florida six weeks later.

The notion of chaos theory was of immediate interest to homeopaths who routinely use extremely dilute solutions in their practice. If a butterfly's wings can cause a hurricane, then what is to stop a very dilute solution of medicine from curing a patient? This is a rather bizarre claim, though, because chaos theory shows the basic unpredictably of nonlinear processes, which is in direct opposition to the claim that homeopathy provides consistently good health outcomes. As Robert Park puts it:

> Thus, while the flapping of a butterfly's wings might conceivably trigger a hurricane, killing butterflies is unlikely to reduce the incidence of hurricanes. As for homeopathic remedies that exceed the dilution limit, a better analogy might be to the flapping of a caterpillar's wings.

Beware of any mechanism that invokes obscure theories in mathematics or physics.

4.10 Summary—What do the other witnesses say?

Be sure to look at all the evidence before making a decision about the persuasiveness of a research study.

Was there a strong association? A strong association reduces the chances that small flaws could invalidate the research.

Was there a dose-response pattern? A dose response rules out some possible biasing factors that would affect all doses uniformly.

Was the association consistent? Replication across a wide range of patients and with a variety of different research designs eliminates a single common flaw as the alternate explanation of the common findings.

Was the association specific? A treatment that shows an effect targeted to a particular outcome reassures you that a global bias in the health of the control group could not produce this result.

Was there a sound biological basis for these findings? A credible mechanism provides additional support for a research finding.

Was there a conflict of interest? When the authors have a financial stake in a particular outcome, they may consciously or subconsciously skew the research findings.

Was there any evidence of fraud? Although fraud is impossible for the reader to detect, a careful review process provides some protection against deliberate falsification of the data.

4.11   On your own

1. Review the following abstract. What corroborating evidence can you find in the abstract itself? Is there a plausible scientific mechanism that would explain how various aspects of the domestic environment might cause snoring problems?

Snoring in primary school children and domestic environment: a Perth school–based study. Zhang, G., Spickett J., Rumchev K., Lee A.H., and Stick S. *Respiratory Research* 2004, 5(1): 19.

Background: The home is the predominant environment for exposure to many environmental irritants such as air pollutants and allergens. Exposure to common indoor irritants including volatile organic compounds, formaldehyde and nitrogen dioxide, may increase the risk of snoring for children. The aim of this study was to investigate domestic environmental factors associated with snoring in children. **Methods:** A school-based respiratory survey was administered during March and April of 2002. Nine hundred and 96 children from four primary schools within the Perth metropolitan area were recruited for the study. A subgroup of 88 children aged 4–6 years were further selected from this sample for domestic air pollutant assessment. **Results:** The prevalence of infrequent snoring and habitual snoring in primary school children were 24.9% and 15.2% respectively. Passive smoking was found to be a significant risk factor for habitual snoring (odds ratio (OR) = 1.77; 95% confidence interval (CI): 1.20–2.61), while having pets at home appeared to be protective against habitual snoring (OR = 0.58; 95% CI: 0.37–0.92). Domestic

pollutant assessments showed that the prevalence of snoring was significantly associated with exposure to nitrogen dioxide during winter. Relative
to the low exposure category (<30 μg/m^3), the adjusted ORs of snoring by
children with medium (30–60 μg/m^3) and high exposures (>60 μg/m^3) to
NO2 were 2.5 (95% CI: 0.7–8.7) and 4.5 (95% CI: 1.4–14.3) respectively.
The corresponding linear dose-response trend was also significant ($p =
0.011$). **Conclusion:** Snoring is common in primary school children. Do-
mestic environments may play a significant role in the increased prevalence
of snoring. Exposure to nitrogen dioxide in domestic environment is associated with snoring in children.

2. In Rosenbaum (2001), three examples are cited where subjects with
ionizing radiation exposure had a higher incidence of leukemia than a
control group.

- Radiologists (who have a high level of exposure to X-rays);
- Patients with ankylosing spondylitis (a condition that is treated with large
  doses of X-rays);
- Survivors of the atomic bombs in Hiroshima and Nagasaki.

For each individual finding, discuss some possible flaws or biases
that might artificially create a relationship between ionizing radiation and
leukemia. Is there a commom flaw?

3. Here are the competing interests that David Sackett lists in the *British
Medical Journal*:

> **Competing interests:** David Sackett has been wined, dined, supported,
> transported, and paid to speak by countless pharmaceutical firms for
> over 40 years, beginning with two research fellowships and interest-free
> loans that allowed him to stay to finish medical school. Dozens of his
> randomized trials have been supported in part (but never in whole) by
> pharmaceutical firms, who have never received or analyzed primary
> data and never had power of veto over any reports, presentations, or
> publications of the results. He has twice worked as a paid consultant to
> advise pharmaceutical firms whether their products caused lethal side
> effects; on both occasions he told them 'yes'. He has testified as an
> unpaid expert witness for a patient who sued a manufacturer of oral
> contraceptives after having a stroke and as a paid expert in preparing a
> class action suit against a manufacturer of prosthetic heart valves. He
> was paid by a pharmaceutical firm to develop 'levels of evidence' for
> determining the causation of adverse drug reactions. His wife inherited
> and sold stock in a pharmaceutical company. While head of a division of
> medicine he enforced the banning of drug detail personnel from clinical
> teaching units (despite the threat of withdrawal of drug industry funding
> for residents' research projects). He received the Pharmaceutical Manu-
> facturers' Association of Canada Medal of Honour (and cash) for
> 'contributions to medical science in Canada' for the decade 1984–94.
> His most recent award (the 2001 Senior Investigator Award of the

Canadian Society of Internal Medicine) was sponsored by Merck Frosst Canada. Posted at bmj.bmjjournals.com/cgi/content/full/324/7336/539/DC1

Which of these interests might be relevant in the editorial he co–authored?

- **Guidelines for managing raised blood pressure.** Jackson, R.T. and Sackett D.L., *British Medical Journal* 1996, 313(7049): 64–5.

5 Do the Pieces Fit Together? Systematic Overviews and Meta-analyses

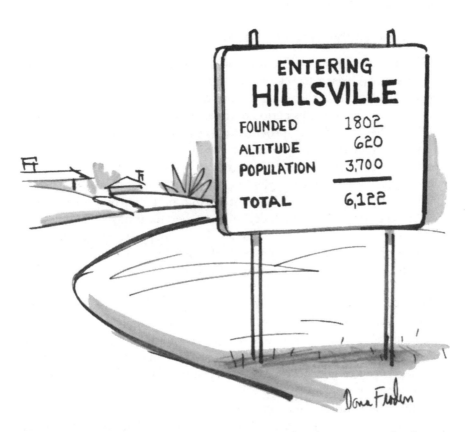

5.1 Introduction

When there are multiple research studies evaluating a new intervention, you need to find a way to assess the cumulative evidence of these studies. You can do this informally, but medical researchers now use a formal process, known as meta-analysis. Meta-analysis, involves the quantitative pooling of data from two or more studies. More recently, another term, systematic overview, has come into favor. A systematic overview involves the careful review and identification of all research studies associated with a topic, but it may or may not end up pooling the results of these studies. So meta-analysis represents a subset of all the systematic overviews. I tend to use the older term, meta-analysis, partly because I am stubborn, but partly because I am interested in the quantitative aspects of this type of research. But most of my comments apply more broadly to systematic overviews.

5.1.1   Case study: Declining sperm counts

In 1992, the *British Medical Journal* published a controversial meta-analysis. This study (Carlsen 1992) reviewed 61 papers published from 1938 and 1991 and showed that there was a significant decrease in sperm count and in seminal volume over this period of time. For example, a linear regression model on the pooled data provided an estimated average count of 113 million per ml in 1940 and 66 million per ml in 1990.

Several researchers (Olsen 1995; Fisch 1996) noted heterogeneity in this meta-analysis, a mixing of apples and oranges. Studies before 1970 were dominated by studies in the United States and particularly studies in New York. Studies after 1970 included many other locations including third world countries. Thus the early studies were US apples. The later studies were international oranges. There was also substantial variation in collection methods, especially in the extent to which the subjects adhered to a minimum abstinence period.

The original meta-analysis and the criticisms of it highlight both the greatest weakness and the greatest strength of meta-analysis.

Meta-analysis is the quantitative pooling of data from studies with sometimes small and sometimes large disparities. Think of it as a multicenter trial where each center gets to use its own protocol and where some of the centers are left out.

On the other hand, a meta-analysis lays all the cards on the table. Sitting out in the open are all the methods for selecting studies, abstracting information, and combining the findings. Meta-analysis allows objective criticism of these overt methods and even allows replication of the research.

Contrast this to an invited editorial or commentary that provides a subjective summary of a research area. Even when the subjective summary is done well, you cannot effectively replicate the findings. Since a subjective review is a black box, the only way, it seems, to repudiate a subjective summary is to attack the messenger.

5.1.2   Do the pieces fit together? What to look for

When you are examining the results of a meta-analysis, you should ask the following questions.

Were apples combined with oranges? Heterogeneity among studies may make any pooled estimate meaningless.

Were some apples left on the tree? An incomplete search of the literature can bias the findings of a meta-analysis.

Were all of the apples rotten? The quality of a meta-analysis cannot be any better than the quality of the studies it is summarizing.

Did the pile of apples amount to more than just a hill of beans? Make sure that the meta-analysis quantifies the size of the effect in units that you can understand.

5.2   Were apples combined with oranges?

Meta-analyses should not have too broad an inclusion criteria. Including too many studies can lead to problems with apples-to-oranges comparisons.

Example: In a meta-analysis looking at antiretroviral combination therapy (Jordan 2002), both short-term and long-term outcomes were examined. A plot of duration of trial versus the log odds ratio showed that shorter duration trials of zidovudine had substantial evidence of effect (odds ratios much smaller than 1) but that the largest duration studies had little or no evidence of effect (odds ratios very close to 1).

Example: In a meta-analysis looking at dust mite control measures to help asthmatic patients (Gotzsche 1998), the studies exhibited heterogeneity across several factors. Six studies examined chemical interventions, thirteen examined physical interventions, and four examined a combination approach. Nine of these trials were crossovers, and in the remaining fourteen, there was a parallel control group. Seven studies had no blinding, three studies had partial blinding, and the remaining thirteen studies used a double blind. In nine studies the average age of the patients was only 9 or 10 years, but nine other studies had an average age of 30 or more. Eleven studies lasted eight weeks or less and five studies lasted a full year.

There is a lot of variability in how research is conducted. Even in carefully controlled randomized trials, researchers have tremendous discretion. This discretion leads to substantial disparities. These disparities create heterogeneity, making it difficult to combine the studies. A review of why randomized trials differ from one another (Horwitz 1987) is instructive. This publication actually predates most of the work in meta-analysis, but still provides a useful guideline for how heterogeneity can occur. The reasons why research studies differ are listed below.

5.2.1   Heterogeneity in the composition of the treatment and control groups

- Researchers can differ in the inclusion and exclusion criteria.

- Even if these criteria do not differ, there may still be differences in the baseline levels of health in the patients, due to geographical differences in the patient population.
- The controls could be selected independently, or they could be matched to the treatment group subjects.
- The control subjects could be given no treatment, a placebo, or a standard treatment.
- The treatment could differ, such as differences in dose or timing of a drug.

5.2.2   Heterogeneity in the design of the study

- The length of follow-up for the patients could differ.
- The proportion of patients who drop out could differ as well as the proposed statistical treatment of these dropouts.

5.2.3   Heterogeneity in the management of the patients and in the outcome

- Patients could differ in how their co-morbid conditions or complications are treated.
- Physicians may have greater or lesser amounts of discretion in the control of their patients' care, such as the ability to adjust dosages of the study drug.

The outcome measure itself could differ. For example, a methodology paper on meta-analysis (Abramson 1990) cited a review of hypertension treatment in the elderly, where some of the studies examined cardiovascular deaths and others examined cardiovascular events.[1] Other studies examined cerebrovascular deaths, cerebrovascular events, cardiac deaths, coronary heart disease deaths, and/or total deaths. The distinctions in the outcome measures are sometime subtle and sometimes not, but they all represent different outcome measures.

5.2.4   How to measure heterogeneity

There is a statistic, Cochran's Q, which provides a numeric measure of heterogeneity. When Q is roughly equal to the number of studies in the meta-analysis, there is little evidence of heterogeneity. When Q is much larger than the number of studies, then you have significant evidence of heterogeneity. There is a similar measure, I-squared, which is based on Cochran's Q (Higgins 2003). I-squared ranges between 0 and 100%. It represents the proportion of variation among the studies that is caused by

---

[1] I'm not quite sure what an 'event' is but I suspect it involves something like a visit to the emergency room. I would much rather suffer a cardiovascular event than a cardiovascular death.

heterogeneity. Small values (25% or less) for I-squared imply that hetero-geneity accounts for little or none of the variation between studies. Larger values, like 50% or 75%, imply that heterogeneity is a serious problem.

Many researchers prefer not to use any quantitative measure of heterogen-eity because these measures do not seem to identify cases where heterogeneity is very large (Gavaghan 2000). Instead, these researchers advocate a qualita-tive examination of heterogeneity by looking at specific study characteristics.

A forest plot can also provide visual evidence of heterogeneity. A forest plot shows each individual study estimate (represented by a square) and confidence limits (represented as lines extending from the square to the upper and lower limits). The size of the square represents the weight that each study receives. There are many ways in which heterogeneity can manifest itself, but you should be especially watchful for one or two outlying studies (e.g. most studies show a strong effect but two show no effect or even a change in the opposite direction). Do not worry, of course, if the outlying studies have very small sample sizes, since these studies would be expected to have a lot of inaccuracy and imprecision. Also watch for an obvious bimodal pattern in the individual study estimates, such as half of the studies showing no effect and the other half showing a strong effect of treatment, with little or no intermediate studies.

Example: In a study of contrast-induced nephropathy after intravascular angiography (Bagshaw 2004), the odds ratios for the effectiveness of prophylactic acetylcysteine plus hydration versus hydration alone are dis-played in a forest plot, as shown below. Odds ratios less than 1 represent findings in favor of acetylcysteine. These odds ratios in this plot show a reasonable amount of consistency, which is evidence that there is little or no heterogeneity. There is some variation in the odds ratios, but they exhibit a range of effects from no effect to a strong effect in favor of the treatment, and some intermediate values as well (see Figure 5.1).

Another approach, the L'Abbe plot, shows the degree of heterogeneity in the placebo response rate. In this plot, the horizontal axis shows the percentage of patients with placebo who show a successful outcome. A similar percentage for the treatment group appears on the vertical axis. A diagonal line separates the plot into two regions, the region lower and to the right represents studies where the percentage is higher in the placebo group. The region higher and to the left represents studies where the percentage is higher in the treatment group. The circles in this plot have diameters that are proportional to the sample size of the individual studies.

When you see this type of plot, examine whether the superiority of the treatment group is uniform across low and high placebo response rates. Studies with a high placebo response rate (those on the right half of the graph), may represent situations where the patients were not very ill to begin with, because even a placebo cures most of them. These studies may

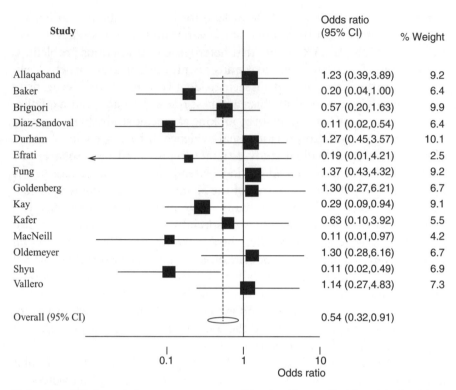

Figure 5.1   This image is from an open source publication. You can find the original article at www.biomedcentral.com/1741-7015/2/38 and this particular figure at www.biomedcentral.com/1741-7015/2/38/figure/F2.

contribute to heterogeneity, because it may be impossible for even a very good treatment to show superiority over a high placebo response rate.

Example: In a meta-analysis of topical NSAIDs for musculoskelatal pain (Mason 2004), the proportion of patients with at least a 50% reduction in pain was plotted for both the placebo group and the NSAID group. All of the studies seem to support the superiority of NSAIDs, though some studies are stronger than others. The key finding, though is that the superiority of NSAIDs persists across the studies, even though the placebo ranged from very low (10%) to very high (80%). This reassures you that there is no serious problem with heterogeneity in spite of a wide range of placebo response rates (see Figure 5.2).

5.2.5   How to handle heterogeneity

Some level of heterogeneity is acceptable. After all, the purpose of research is to generalize results to large groups of patients. Furthermore, demonstrating that a treatment shows consistent results across a variety of conditions strengthens our confidence in that treatment. Nevertheless, you should

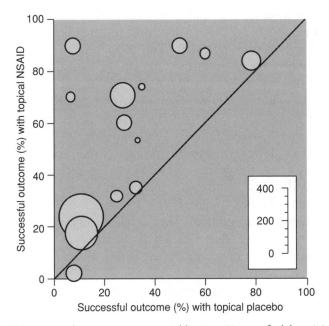

Figure 5.2   This image is from an open source publication. You can find the original article at www.biomedcentral.com/1471-2474/5/28 and this particular figure at www.biomedcentral.com/1471-2474/5/28/figure/F1.

be aware of the problems that excessive heterogeneity can cause. Mixing apples and oranges may not be so bad; you get a fruit salad this way. But when heterogeneity becomes too large, you might end up combining not apples and oranges but apples and onions.

One way to handle heterogeneity is to be very restrictive in the types of studies that you choose. Meta-analyses should not have too broad an inclusion criteria. For example, when you are studying the effect of cholesterol lowering drugs, it makes no sense to combine a study of patients with recent heart attacks (secondary prevention) with another study of patients with high cholesterol but no previous heart attacks (primary prevention).

Example: In a meta-analysis of topical NSAIDs for musculoskelatal pain (Mason 2004), identified 60 target papers, but for 12 of the papers, there was no data that could be extracted for a meta-analysis. An additional 23 studies were removed based on the following exclusion criteria:

- no studies for mouth or eye diseases;
- no studies where fewer than 10 patients were randomized to the treatment;
- no studies where treatment occurred less frequently than daily;
- no observational studies; and
- no unblinded studies.

Placing a time limit on the studies to be included can also help. It does depend on the topic being studied, but most research that is more than two decades old is probably irrelevant. This is especially true in a field like neonatology where the babies being successfully rescued keep getting smaller and smaller.

Example: In a systematic overview of proton pump inhibitors for the treatment of acute ulcers (Salas 2002), the researchers selected only those papers appearing between January 1990 and July 2001. The researchers also excluded any long-term treatments (greater than six months).

Other areas where the practice of medicine has been much more stable could have wider time windows. I have seen several reviews that have covered half a century of studies. If you do select a wide time window, be sure to see whether your results are similar when you restrict yourself to just the most recent studies. Ask yourself if there was a sudden change in technology that makes any comparisons before and after that technology an apples-to-oranges comparison.

AIDS patients represent a group where the time window is very important. When this disease first appeared, there was no treatment for it and diagnosis of AIDS was effectively a death sentence. But around 1987, new drugs, starting with AZT, became available, and while they do not cure the disease, they allow people to live with the disease. So any meta-analysis involving AIDS patients should restrict itself to the years following the use of AZT.

5.2.6 Sensitivity analysis

A good approach to heterogeneity is to include a wide range of studies, but then to examine the sensitivity of the results by looking at more narrowly drawn subsets of the studies.

Example: In a study of extra corporeal shock wave therapy for plantar heel pain (Thomson 2005), six studies met the researchers inclusion criteria, but one study did not report a standard deviation for the outcome measure. The authors were forced to estimate what the standard deviation should be for this study. As a quality check, they also ran a meta-analysis without this study and found that a modest effect in favor of the therapy was no longer statistically significant.

Example: In a study of topical NSAIDs for osteoarthritis and tendinitis (Mason 2004), researchers identified 25 trials relating to efficacy or harm and separated the trials into placebo-controlled trials and trials where the control group got a comparison drug rather than placebo. It makes sense to analyze the placebo trials separately, because you would expect those trials to have a much larger effect. The 14 placebo controlled trials for efficacy varied substantially in their quality scores, the number of patients studied, the type of outcome measure (physician determined versus self report) and the condition being treated (osteoarthritis versus other musculoskeletal conditions). But when the results were tabulated separately for low and high quality scores, small and large studies, etc., there were no statistically significant differences.

Example: In a meta-analysis studying atypical antipsychotics (Geddes 2000), the dose of the comparison drug (haloperidol or an equivalent) varied substantially. Among those studies where the dose of haloperidol was greater than 12 mg/day, atypical antipsychotics showed advantages in efficacy or tolerability. When the dose was less than or equal to 12 mg/day, the atypical antipsychotics showed no advantages in these areas.

These sensitivity analyses seem a lot like the subgroup analyses that I had criticized in Chapter 3. Sensitivity analysis does indeed increase the number of comparisons that are being made, but typically, these comparisons are intended as a quality check rather than as a primary outcome of the research.

5.2.7   Meta-regression

You can use meta-regression to try to adjust for heterogeneity in a meta-analysis. In meta-regression, each study becomes a data point, and various study characteristics, such as the severity of illness at baseline, the dose of the medication being given, etc. become independent variables. This is an approach that would work very similarly to the adjustment for covariates in a regression model. The result, meta-regression, is an area of active research and looks to be a promising way to handle heterogeneity in a more rigorous fashion.

Example: In a meta-analysis examining if long-term aspirin therapy was associated with problems with gastrointestinal hemorrhage (Derry 2000), researchers identified 24 studies that looked at aspirin as a preventive measure against heart attacks. In each of these studies, the rate of gastrointestinal hemorrhages were recorded for both the aspirin group and the placebo or no-treatment group. There was substantial heterogeneity in the dosage of aspirin used in the studies, however, with some studies giving as little as 50 mg/day and some as much as 1,500 mg/day. This was actually good news in a way, because the researchers wanted to see if the risk of gastrointestinal hemorrhage was dependent on the dose of aspirin. A plot of the dose versus the risk showed that there was indeed an increased risk among all aspirin users compared to the control group, but this risk seemed to be unrelated to the dosage.

Example: In a study of diagnostic tests for endometrial hyperplasia (Clark 2004), researchers identified 27 studies using miniature endometrial biopsy devices or ultrasonography. In some of the studies, verification of the diagnosis was delayed by more than 24 hours. Although the ability to discriminate between diseased and healthy patients was present in most studies, the discriminatory power, as measured by the diagnostic odds ratio was four times weaker among studies with delayed verification than studies with no delay.

5.2.8   Just say no

If the degree of heterogeneity is too extreme, you should just say no and refuse to run a meta-analysis. You can still discuss the studies in a qualitative fashion, but do not try to compute an overall estimate of effect because that estimate would be meaningless.

Example: In a systematic review of beta-2 agonists for treating chronic obstructive pulmonary disease (Husereau 2004), researchers identified 12 studies. But the authors could not pool the results because they

> found that even commonly measured outcomes, such as FEV1, could not be combined by meta-analysis because of differences in how they were reported. For example, in the six trials comparing salmeterol with placebo, FEV1 was reported as a mean change in percent predicted, a mean change overall, a mean difference between trial arms, no difference (without data), baseline and overall FEV1 (after 24 hrs without medication) and as an 0 to 12 hour area-under-the-curve (FEV1-AUC) function. We were not successful in obtaining more data from study authors. We also had concerns about the meta-analysis of data from trials of parallel and crossover design and differences in spirometry protocols including allowable medications. Therefore, we decided on a best evidence synthesis approach instead.

5.2.9   Heterogeneity: What to look for

In general, heterogeneity increases uncertainty, but this uncertainty cannot be reflected in the width of the confidence limits in the meta-analysis results. When there is heterogeneity, the most information may reside not in a single estimate of how effective the treatment is, but in a careful examination of the variation in the treatment under different conditions.

5.3   Were some apples left on the tree?

One of the greatest concerns in a meta-analysis is whether all the relevant studies have been identified. If some studies are missed, this could lead to serious biases.

5.3.1   Publication bias

Many important studies are never published; these studies are more likely to be negative (Dickersin 1990). This is known as publication bias. Publication bias is the tendency on the parts of investigators, reviewers, and editors to submit or accept manuscripts for publication based on the direction or strength of the study findings. Prevention of publication bias is important both from the scientific perspective (complete dissemination of knowledge) and from the perspective of those who combine results from a number of similar studies (meta-analysis).

Perhaps this is not too surprising. Researchers with a positive finding might fight harder for publication, trying a second or third journal in the face of rejection. With a negative study, they might just give up after one unfavorable review and invest their time somewhere else.

Researchers who fail to publish their research, however, are behaving unethically (Chalmers 1990). These research studies almost always use human volunteers. These volunteers might be participating because they need the money or perhaps they are curious about the scientific process. But many of them volunteer because they want to help others who have the same disease or condition. These volunteers submit themselves willingly to some level of inconvenience, and possibly additional pain and risk. If you ask these volunteers to make this sacrifice, but you do not publish, you have abused their good will.

The inclusion of unpublished studies, however, is controversial. At least one reference (Cook 1993), has argued that unpublished studies have failed to meet a basic quality screen, the peer review process. Including studies that have not been peer reviewed will lower the overall quality of the meta-analysis. This opinion, however, is in the minority, and most experts in meta-analysis suggest that you include unpublished studies if you can find them.

Another aspect of publication bias is that the delay in publication of negative results is likely to be longer than that for positive studies. For example, among 130 clinical trials, the median time to publication was 4.7 years among the positive studies and 8.0 years among the negative studies (Stern 1997). So a meta-analysis restricted to a certain time window may be more likely to exclude published research that is negative.

5.3.2 Duplicate publication

Duplicate publication is the flip side of the publication bias coin. Studies that are positive are more likely to appear more than once in publication. This is especially problematic for multicenter trials where individual centers may publish results specific to their site.

Example: In 84 studies of the effect of ondansetron on postoperative emesis, 14 (17%) were second or even third time publications of the same data-set (Tramer 1997). The duplicate studies had much larger effects and adding the duplicates to the originals produced an overestimation of treatment efficacy of 23%. Tracking down the duplicate publications was quite difficult. More than 90% of the duplicate publications did not cross-reference the other studies. Four pairs of identical trials were published by completely different authors without any common authorship.

Duplicate publication also raises serious ethical issues. First, most researchers offer copyright to the journals they publish in as a condition of research. To republish these results somewhere else without getting permission is a violation of that copyright. Second, these researchers are padding their resumé to make themselves look more attractive for promotion and/or for research grant committees. Third, these researchers are abusing a review system that relies on volunteers to provide peer review. Fourth, they are taking space in a journal for their redundant publications that could have been used for another study.

There are some exceptions that represent legitimate duplicate publications. A study might publish short-term outcomes quickly and then might publish long-term outcomes in a later publication. Sometimes an important result in a non-English language journal gets translated and republished in an English language journal. The main difference with these legitimate practices is that the duplication is clearly acknowledged. The unethical duplicate publications, in contrast, are done covertly, making it much more difficult for anyone conducting a meta-analysis to use these findings.

5.3.3   The limitations of a Medline search

The first place that most researchers search for information is Medline. Medline is a database of over 15 million articles published between 1966 and today in over 4,800 medical journals. Medline also includes a limited number of publications before 1966. The Medline database is maintained by the National Library of Medicine in the US National Institutes of Health. There are several commercial vendors who offer the ability to search through Medline, and you can also search through Medline for free at pubmed.gov.

While a Medline search is a very effective way to identify published research, it should not be the only source of publications for a meta-analysis. There are many important journals which are not included in Medline. It is hard to get an accurate count of how many journals do not appear in Medline, but the numbers appear to be substantial.[2] You might suspect that journals indexed by Medline are more prestigious and more likely to publish positive findings than other journals, but I am unaware of any data to substantiate this. Still, a search that included only Medline articles would be considered grossly inadequate in most situations.

---

[2] One source (www.sl.nsw.gov.au/databases/his.cfm) compiles a database 'for over a hundred Australian health and medical journals not indexed by Medline'. It also appears that journals from India are substantially underrepresented in Medline (Egger 1998).

5.3.4 Using only English language publications

Some meta-analyses restrict their attention to English language publications only. While this may seem like a convenience, in some situations, researchers might tend to publish in an English language journal for those trials which are positive, and publish in a (presumably less prestigious) native language journal for those trials which are negative (Gregoire 1995).

Restriction to English language only publications is especially troublesome for complementary and alternative medicine, since so much of this research appears in non-English language journals. But it is a troublesome restriction for any meta-analysis. I have only seen one exception to this rule. Researchers were trying to identify studies of adverse drug reactions in the United States (Lazarou 1998) so they could estimate the number of patient deaths associated with this problem. When you are interested only in deaths that occur in the United States, it seems reasonable to believe that all of the available research would have been published in English.

5.3.5 Picking the low hanging fruit

In an informal meta-analysis, you should also worry about the tendency for people to preferentially choose articles that are convenient. For example, there is a natural tendency to rely on articles where the full text is available on the Internet or where the abstract is available for review (Wentz 2002). I am fortunate. When I select examples for this book or for my web pages, I can deliberately target those journals with full free text. A research paper that is easy for me to get is a useful teaching tool because it is also easy for my readers to get. But a practicing clinician cannot afford to limit his or her attention to papers that are within easy reach.

5.3.6 Subjective exclusion

Like any other research project, an overview or meta-analysis needs a protocol. The protocol should specify (among other things) the inclusion/exclusion criteria for studies. These standards should be as objective as possible, but there will always be some level of subjectivity. Authors have been shown to be biased in the articles that they cite in the bibliographies of their research papers (Gotzsche 1987; Ravnskov 1992). This same bias could potentially affect the selection of articles in a meta-analysis. The researcher may consciously or subconsciously apply the exclusion criteria more strictly for studies that have one type of outcome and more loosely for studies that have the opposite outcome.

One way to avoid subjective application of the exclusion criteria is to use blinding. The people deciding whether a paper should be in the meta-analysis should be unaware of the authors of that paper and the journal.

They should also include or exclude the paper on the basis of the methods section only; they should not see the results section until later. There is empirical evidence, however, that blinding does not affect the conclusions of a meta-analysis (Jadad 1996; Berlin 1997). Furthermore, blinding takes substantial time and energy. In my opinion, blinding is nice to have because you have extra insurance against claims of bias.

Data should be extracted from papers by two independent reviewers and their level of agreement should be assessed. Researchers should also list all of the articles found in the original search, not just the articles used. This allows others to examine whether the inclusion/exclusion criteria were applied appropriately.

For all of the efforts to make meta-analysis an objective and repeatable process, some level of human subjectivity is unavoidable. In a Cochrane Database System Review of mammography (Olsen 2001), seven studies were identified, but only two were of sufficient quality to be used. The Cochrane Review of these two studies reached a negative conclusion, but would have reached an opposite conclusion if the other five studies were added back in (Mayor 2001). Which analysis is correct? There is no obvious answer because there is no authority you can appeal to who could tell you inerrantly what studies to include/exclude.

5.3.7   Detecting publication bias

The most common approach to evaluate publication bias is to use a funnel plot. The funnel plot displays the results of the individual studies (e.g. the log odds ratio) on the horizontal axis, and the size of the study (or sometimes the standard error of the study) on the vertical axis. Often a reference line is drawn at the value that represents no effect to visually separate the region where the new treatment is considered more effective from the region where the standard treatment (or placebo) is considered more effective. The rationale behind this plot is that the big studies get published no matter what the result. If you have invested the time and money to study thousands of patients, you will work equally hard to get the result published. Among smaller studies, though, you may preferentially work harder to publish the positive findings.

If there is no publication bias, then the funnel plot should show symmetry for both small sample sizes and large sample sizes, though you should expect to see less variation as the sample size increases. This leads to a funnel shape. A deviation from a symmetric funnel shape indicates the possibility of publication bias, especially if there are very few studies with a small sample size in the region where the standard treatment appears to be more effective.

Example: In a study of contrast-induced nephropathy (Bagshaw 2004), researchers found 14 studies looking at acetylcysteine as a treatment for this

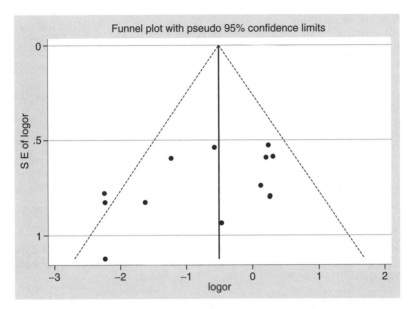

Figure 5.3   This image is from an open source publication. You can find the original article at www.biomedcentral.com/1741-7015/2/38 and this particular figure at www.biomedcentral. com/1741-7015/2/38/figure/F4.

condition. A funnel plot showed a roughly symmetric distribution of studies, which is evidence that publication bias is not a serious problem here (see Figure 5.3).

Example: In a study of oral rehydration (Bellemare 2004), researchers found 14 trials comparing this treatment to intravenous therapy. A funnel plot of these studies shows a lack of symmetry and the direction of the asymmettry indicates that the unpublished studies might have a greater tendency to favor oral rehydration (see Figure 5.4).

The problem with the funnel plot is that there is no standardized way to draw the plot (Tang 2000) and interpretation of the funnel plot is subjective. Furthermore, an asymmetric pattern might just be a reflection of the poorer quality that occurs more often in small studies (Sterne 2001). There are several quantitative measures based on the funnel plot but these may also be difficult to interpret.

An alternative to the funnel plot is a sensitivity analysis. You would compare the articles that were easy to find (e.g. in Medline) with those that were hard to find (e.g. results presented at a meeting but never published). If there is no discrepancy between the easy to find and the hard to find articles, then perhaps you can extrapolate and say that there is probably no difference between the easy to find articles and the articles that you never did find.

Another type of sensitivity analysis is to estimate the number of undiscovered negative studies that would be required to overturn the results of

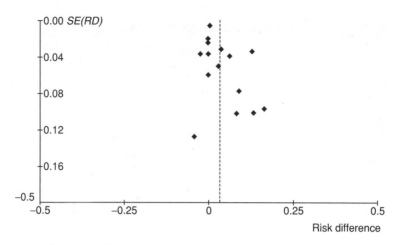

Figure 5.4   This image is from an open source publication. You can find the original article at www.biomedcentral.com/1741-7015/2/11 and this particular figure at www.biomedcentral.com/1741-7015/2/11/figure/F3.

this meta-analysis. If the number of undiscovered negative studies is just two, then you should be cautious, but if the number were 500, then you could rest assured that the positive finding was almost certainly not caused by publication bias.

   Example: In a study of patients with variceal hemorrhage (Corley 2001), researchers identifed 13 studies comparing octerotide, a syntehtic hormone, to a variety of alternative treatments (vasopressin/terlipressin, placebo, or sclerotherapy). The overall effect of octerotide compared to all alternatives combines in sustained control of bleeding was statistically significant. The relative risk was 0.58 (95% CI 0.51–0.77) and the number needed to treat was 8 (95% CI 5–16). The authors estimated that it would take 31 unpublished negative studies to nullify this result. This number is large (especially considering that only 13 total studies were identified) which gives you substantial reassurance that publication bias did not, by itself, produce this result.

5.3.8   How to avoid bias from exclusion of publications

Search for studies should involve *several* bibliographic databases. Additional databases include CINAHL (the Cumulative Index to Nursing and Allied Health Literature) that focuses on articles relating to nursing and allied health. CINAHL covers 1,200 nursing and allied health journals since 1982. EMBASE is a database with extensive coverage of pharmacological data. EMBASE includes many European and Asian journals not covered by Medline. EMBASE currently has 16 million articles and covers over 6,000 journals.

   You should also look for searches that include registries for clinical trials. A registry is a voluntary system for researchers to document the existence of their clinical trials. Typically, this can (and should) be done at the start of the research study so there is no possibility that the outcome of the study could influence registration.

If you expect some of the publications to appear in specialized journals, then you might want to hand search the table of contents for all of these journals. For example, a meta-analysis of prophylactic antibiotics in children at risk for urinary tract infection might review the last ten years of Pediatric Nephrology.

The Cochrane Collaboration also maintains several registries of clinical trials. Volunteers regularly search through the published literature using established search methods to find research articles relating to particular topics. For example, you can search a Cochrane registry of trials in Complementary and Alternative Medicine at www.compmed.umm.edu/Cochrane/Registry.html.

A search should also look at the bibliographies of all articles found on the first pass through to try to identify any additional studies not identified elsewhere.

A search should also include the 'gray literature': presentation abstracts, dissertations, theses, etc. Researchers can also send out a letter to prominent experts in the field calling for information about unpublished research.

Example: In a study of near patient testing, tests where the results are available without sending materials to a lab (McManus 1998), the authors used a search of electronic databases, a survey of experts in the area, and hand searching of specific journals. The electronic databases yielded the most number of publications, 50, but still missed 52 publications found by the other two methods.

Example: In a study of air travel and deep vein thrombosis (Adi 2004), the following search strategy was used:

> Using a combination of text words and MeSH headings, MEDLINE, EMBASE, Cochrane databases (CDSR, CENTRAL) and National Research Register (NRR) were searched using the search strategy shown in Appendix 1 [see Additional file 1]. Citations of included studies and reviews were checked, and experts in the field were contacted. Two types of studies were sought: incidence rate from longitudinal studies and comparative studies to estimate the risk of DVT (i.e. the risk of DVT in air travellers relative to non air travellers).

5.3.9 Correcting for publication bias

Correcting for publication bias is very controversial because it involves extrapolating through the inclusion of a group of unseen studies of uncertain results.

Example: A re-analysis of a meta-analysis on lung cancer (Copas 2000) adjusted for publication bias. They noticed a lack of symmetry in a plot similar to a funnel plot and also noted a modest correlation (0.35) between the uncertainty of a study and the effect shown. As the uncertainty increased, the effect increased as well. If there were no correlation, then there would be no evidence that small negative studies remain unpublished. The researchers then estimated the relative risk by assuming that there were an additional 10%, 20%, 30%, and 40% unpublished negative studies and estimated what would have happened if these studies were found. The relative risk of smoking declined from 1.24 to 1.18, 1.15, 1.13, and 1.11 respectively. The authors admitted, however, that there was no good way to estimate the number of unpublished studies. Several criticisms of this approach were published (Johnson 2000; Hackshaw 2000; Glantz 2000; Cates 2000).

The trim-and-fill method takes the actual funnel plot and adds a limited number pseudo-studies to force the plot to be symmetric. Then this method computes an adjusted estimate controlling for publication bias by estimating the overall effect with the inclusion of the extra pseudo-studies. The idea of imputing extra studies and adding them to an analysis might make you uncomfortable. It does have the appearance of just manufacturing data, but it is worth noting that statisticians will often impute values in a randomized trial where some of the patients drop out, so there is some precedent for this type of approach.

Example: In review of 48 meta-analyses published in the Cochrane Database of Systematic Reviews (Sutton 2000), the trim-and-fill method was applied in the 26 studies where there was evidence of publication bias. In four of these analyses, the trim-and-fill method produced a different conclusion. The authors stressed that this approach should not replace the published estimates, but instead be considered as a way to explore the sensitivity of a meta-analysis to publication bias.

5.3.10   Publication bias: What to look for

Omission of unpublished or difficult to find studies could bias the conclusions of the meta-analysis. Look for evidence of a thorough search for relevant publications. Make sure that the authors did not take the easy way out, for example, by limiting the search to only English language publications.

5.4   Were all of the apples rotten?

A homogeneous set of studies is not good if the studies are homogeneously bad. The quality of a meta-analysis is constrained by the quality of articles that are used in a meta-analysis. Meta-analysis cannot correct or compensate for methodologically flawed studies. In fact, meta-analysis may reinforce or amplify the flaws of the original studies.

5.4.1   Observational studies in a meta-analysis

The use of meta-analysis on observational studies is very controversial. Many meta-analyses start off with randomization as part of the inclusion criteria, but others allow nonrandomized studies to participate as well. For some areas, observational studies may be the only studies available.

Is it acceptable to include observational studies in a meta-analysis? A collaborative effort known as MOOSE (meta-analysis of observational studies in epidemiology) provided reporting guidelines to improve the quality of these types of overviews (Stroup 2000). Some experts have argued, however, against including observational studies in a meta-analysis, including one expert who said that such an inclusion makes meta-analysis 'an exercise in mega-silliness' (Eysenck 1978). But even those experts who do not take such an extreme viewpoint warn that the current statistical methods for summarizing the results of observational studies may grossly understate the amount of uncertainty in the final result (Egger 1998).

The theory behind this criticism notes first that observational studies have systematic biases, and there is no easy way to correct for systematic biases in a meta-analysis. Uncertainties associated with small sample sizes cause random variations in either direction, and these cancel out when you combine multiple studies. But uncertainties or biases associated with weak research designs tend to point in the same direction, and these biases are preserved in the meta-analysis. So the relative importance of bias may be moderate in a single small observational study, but it rises to a position of great prominence in a meta-analysis.

If these observational studies represented the exact same type of study, then the meta-analysis would be estimating the systematic bias associated with this type of study. It is a good theory, up to a point, but keep in mind that randomized studies also have sources of bias. Furthermore, the biases inherent in observational studies are not always pointing in the same direction. If the observational studies represent a variety of different designs and approaches, it is less likely that they would all share biases that point in a common direction.

Some meta-analyses restrict their attention to randomized trials because these studies are less likely to have problems with bias. In other words, they wish to avoid mixing bad observational apples with good randomized trial apples. Keep in mind, though, the counterpoint offered in Chapter 1.

There are variations in the quality among observational studies as well. Typically (but not universally), cohort studies produce more credible evidence than case-control studies and prospective studies produce more credible evidence than retrospective studies. Separating out the different types of observational studies may give you clues as to the overall quality of the pooled estimate.

Example: A review of the risk of Alzheimer's disease in users of nonsteroidal anti-inflammatory drugs (Etminan 2003), researchers identified six cohort studies, which showed a combined relative risk of 0.84 (95% CI 0.54–1.05) and three case-control studies which showed a much lower combined relative risk, 0.62 (95% CI 0.45–0.82).

5.4.2 Meta-analysis of studies with small sample sizes

You should be very careful in the assessment of meta-analyses where all of the trials have small sample sizes. The effect of publication bias can be far more pronounced here than in situations where some medium and large size trials are included. In addition, smaller studies tend to have greater problems with the methods of randomizing and blinding patients (Kjaergard 2001).

Example: In a meta-analysis of gastric versus post-pyloric feeding (Marik 2003), researchers identified nine studies that met the inclusion/exclusion criteria. The total number of patients in these studies ranged from 25 to 101 and the total number of subjects across all nine studies was only 552. The researchers noted the small sample sizes in their conclusion and warned that these results should be 'interpreted with some caution'.

5.4.3 Meta-analysis of Chinese studies

Research published in Chinese journals have shown a substantial deficit in quality that should make you cautious about any meta-analysis using these studies. For example, a review of Chinese medicinal herbs in the treatment of hepatitis B (Liu 2002) showed inadequate documentation of the randomization method and failure of most studies to conceal the allocation list. Further, a small fraction of these studies showed a degree of imbalance between the treatment and control that was well beyond what you would expect by chance.

A review article on acupuncture (Vickers 1998) evaluated articles published in various countries. In China, 100% of the acupuncture studies showed a positive result. In areas other than acupuncture, the results were similar. In Chinese journals, 99% of the nonacupuncture studies were positive. To form a basis of comparison, only 75% of the studies published in England were positive. Another revealing statistic was that Chinese journals *never* published a finding to show that the new therapy was less effective than the control group. There were similar problems with publications from Japan, Taiwan, and Russia.

A review of 2,938 publications in Chinese journals (Tang 1999) also noted many problems:

> Although methodological quality has been improving over the years, many problems remain. The method of randomisation was often in-

appropriately described. Blinding was used in only 15% of trials. Only a few studies had sample sizes of 300 subjects or more. Many trials used as a control another Chinese medicine treatment whose effectiveness had often not been evaluated by randomised controlled trials. Most trials focused on short term or intermediate rather than long term outcomes. Most trials did not report data on compliance and completeness of follow up. Effectiveness was rarely quantitatively expressed and reported. Intention to treat analysis was never mentioned.

This paper also shows evidence of serious publication bias. They display a funnel plot for studies of acupuncture for the treatment of stroke, for example, which shows a serious asymmetry with only 3 studies out of 49 showing a negative effect, but a large number of studies, especially studies with small sample sizes lying just above the threshold of no effect (see Figure 5.5).

5.4.4 Rating the quality of the studies

Any effort to control for the quality of research studies needs a way, either quantitative or qualitative, to assess that quality. There are quantitiative measures used in meta-analysis. The Jadad score (Jadad 1996) rates three things:

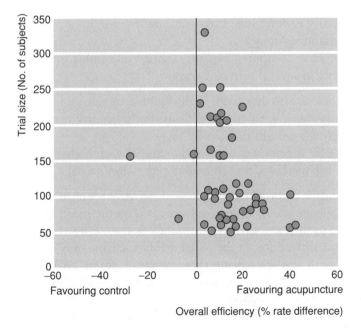

Figure 5.5 A funnel plot of 49 studies of accupuncture, showing serious evidence of publication bias. This figure from Tang et al. BMJ 1999 (July 17) 319: 160–161 and is reproduced with permission from the BMJ Publishing Group.

- Randomization (2 points if method is described well and is appropriate, 1 point if method has no description);
- Blinding (2 points if double blind with good description, 1 point if study is blinded but with no description);
- Withdawals/dropouts (1 point for description of the number of withdrawals and reasons).

Another quality score is the PEDro score (Maher 2003) which is used in physical therapy research. This scale evaluates 11 components:

1. Eligibility criteria were specified.
2. Subjects were randomly allocated to groups (or, in a crossover study, subjects were randomly allocated to an order in which treatments were received).
3. Allocation was concealed.
4. Groups were similar at baseline.
5. Subjects were blinded.
6. Therapists who administered the treatment were blinded.
7. Assessors were blinded.
8. Measures of key outcomes were obtained from more than 85% of subjects.
9. Data were analyzed by intention to treat.
10. Statistical comparisons between groups were conducted.
11. Point measures and measures of variability were provided.

The total score is determined by counting the number of criteria that are satisfied, excluding item 1.

Once you have computed a quality score, you can incorporate it into the meta-analysis in several different ways:

- You can use the quality score in the inclusion/exclusion criteria.
- You can perform a subgroup analysis on the studies with quality scores above/below a certain threshold.
- You can give greater weight to those studies with higher quality.
- You can use quality scores in a meta-regression model.

Example: In a meta-analysis of topical NSAIDs for chronic musculoskeletal pain (Mason 2004), all studies were rated on the Jadad quality scale. To be included in the meta-analysis, the study had to score at least two points on the Jadad scale. Later in the paper, studies scoring only two points were compared with studies scoring three or more points on the Jadad scale. When the low scoring studies were excluded, the pooled estimate of effect did not show a sizable change.

Example: In a study of extra corporeal shock wave therapy for plantar heel pain (Thomson 2005), the researchers computed quality scores for each study and looked at the results for the four studies with high quality scores. The combined effects from those four high quality studies were not statistically significant compared to a statistically significant finding when all six studies were combined.

Many times, the reporting of a study will be incomplete or ambiguous, and this will make it impossible to assess the quality of a study. There is indeed empirical evidence that incomplete reporting is associated with poor quality (Schulz 1995). In such a case, a 'guilty until proven innocent' approach may make sense (Juni 2001). For example, if the authors fail to mention whether their study was blinded, assume that it was not. You might expect that authors would be quick to report strengths of their study, but may (perhaps unconsciously) forget to mention their weaknesses. On the other hand, Liberati (1986) rated the quality of 63 randomized trials, and found that the quality scores increased by seven points on average on a 100 point scale after talking to the researchers over the telephone. So some small amount of ambiguity may relate to carelessness in reporting rather than quality problems.

There is considerable concern about the use of quality scores (Greenland 2001). Do they oversimplify things? Are they valid? This is an area of active research right now, and there are not any well-accepted standards on how to properly account for the quality of the individual studies in a meta-analysis.

5.4.5   Poor quality studies in meta-analysis: What to look for

Meta-analysis cannot make a silk purse out of a sow's ear. If there are serious methodological limitations to the quality of all the studies in a meta-analysis, the meta-analysis itself will have serious limitations. Look for an assessment of quality and a sensitivity analysis that compares the varying levels of quality.

5.5   Did the pile of apples amount to more than just a hill of beans?

It is not enough to know that the overall effect of a therapy is positive. You have to balance the magnitude of the effect versus the added cost and/or the side effects of the new therapy. Is the effect large enough to have a practical impact? Is the final result clinically important?

Example: In a study of the effect of smoking cessation programs on the health of the fetus and infant (Lumley 2000), researchers used birth weight as one of the primary outcomes. The study showed that the typical program can improve birth weight by a statistically significant amount. The researchers then quantified the amount: 28 g (95% confidence interval 9–49). This effect, by itself, is too small to justify the trouble and expense of the smoking cessation program. It's worth noting here that stopping smoking still makes a lot of sense for pregnant women. The small effect seen here is more an indictment of the failure of smoking cessation programs to find ways to help people quit smoking in large numbers.

How do you assess what is clinically important? Start by using the same guidelines on clinical importance in Chapter 3. Beware of surrogate outcomes unless they can be tied to a patient oriented outcome. You should also be cautious about unblinded or retrospective measures. But meta-analysis also has its own unique issues.

5.5.1 Vote counting

Avoid 'vote counting' or the tallying of positive versus negative studies. Vote counts ignore the possibility that some studies are negative solely because of their sample size. As noted in a methodology article on meta-analysis (Abramson 1990), you can show a positive result even when each of the individual studies was negative, as long as most of the studies were pointing in the same general direction. The combination of all of these studies does sometimes show a positive result, proving the Statistician's motto 'There's strength in numbers.'

5.5.2 Unitless measures

When you are examining a continuous outcome measure, you should be sure that the results are presented in interpretable units. Unfortunately, many meta-analyses use an effect size or standardized mean difference (the improvement due to the therapy divided by the standard deviation). The effect size is unitless, allowing the combination of results from studies where slightly different outcomes with slightly different measurement units might have been used.

A measure of effect size, however, does not help you much because it is unitless and impossible to interpret. Consider a store that is offering a sale and announces boldly: 'All prices reduced by 0.8 standard deviations!'

You have no way to know whether this sale provides a lot of savings or just a trivial amount. The same is true for an effect size. To interpret it properly, you need to transform it back into the original scale of measurement.

Example: In a meta-analysis of educational interventions for self-management of asthma (Guevara 2003), four studies had complete data on lung function. This was measured either as change in forced expiratory volume or in peak expiratory flow rate or in percentage predicted peak flow rate. The only way to combine these disparate measures was to standardize them. The pooled result of the standardized measures showed an effect size of 0.5 (95% CI, 0.25–0.75). So the education programs improved lung function by half a standard deviation. The authors were nice enough to transform this back into the original scales. Half a standard deviation corresponds to 0.24 liter increase in forced expiratory volume or a 9.5% increase in percentage of predicted peak flow.

5.5.3 Measures of risk

The most easily interpretable measures of risk are the number needed to treat (NNT) and the number needed to harm (NNH) (see pp. 146–7 for further details). Ideally, the results of a meta-analysis presenting measures like an odds ratio or a relative risk should also be presented in the more readily interpretable NNT/NNH format.

Example: In a study of early postnatal dexamethasone for prevention of chronic lung disease (Bhuta 1998), researchers estimated the number needed to treat for the mortality outcome as 8 (95% CI, 4–30). In other words, you would have to treat 8 patients with dexamethasone in order to see one fewer death. There were similar results for the NNT for prevention of chronic lung disease. The NNH for hypertension was 42 (95% CI 19–212) and for hyperglycemia, it was 14 (95% CI, 8–100).

Unfortunately, there are problems with computing NNT/NNH for each study and then combining them (Smeeth 1999; Cates 2002). These values are highly sensitive to the response rate for the standard treatment/placebo. A better approach would be to estimate a common odds ratio or relative risk, and then calculate the NNT/NNH for a plausible background or placebo response rate.

5.5.4 Meta-analyses of diagnostic studies

The standards for meta-analysis of diagnostic studies are still evolving. A popular approach is to combine the results using a diagnostic odds ratio (DOR). The DOR contrasts the sensitivity and specificity of a study and is largest when both sensitivity and specificity are very close to 100%.

The DOR was suggested as a summary measure to combine results in a meta-analysis of diagnostic studies (Deeks 2001; Deville 2002). It is very useful because some studies may adjust a test to give higher sensitivity at the expense of specificity or vice versa. If you tried to combine all the sensitivities and then separately combine all of the specificities, you would get a mediocre value for both.

Figure 5.6 shows a hypothetical range of sensitivities and specificity as circles. This range reflects the typical trade-off between sensitivity and specificity. If you naively combined the sensitivities and naively combined the specificities, you would get the value represented by the plus sign, a value that underestimates the performance that this diagnostic test is capable of.

The DOR does avoid some of these problems, but like the effect size, is difficult to interpret in practice. What does a DOR of 24 mean? It would be better if the authors gave a practical interpretation that represent what 24 means with respect to a particular sensitivity/specificity pair. One way that you can coneptualize the DOR is to factor it into a pair of odds, one for sensitivity and one for specificity. So, you could allocate an odds of 6 to 1

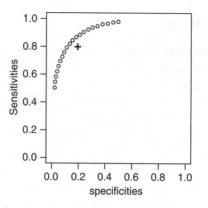

Figure 5.6 Hypothetical range of sensitivities and specificities (circles) and the average (plus sign).

for sensitivity, which corresponds to a probability of 86% and allocate the remaining odds, 4 to 1 for specificity, which translates to a probability of 80%. Alternately, if the test is usually set up to maximize specificity, you could allocate 2 to 1 odds for sensitivity (67%) and 12 to 1 odds for specificity (92%). Unfortunately, if you are like me, you are not comfortable with the concept of odds. It would be better if the authors of the research did this type of calculation for you.

Example: In a study of the urine dipstick test (Deville 2004), the effectiveness of the test was evaluated across several patient groups using a diagnostic odds ratio. In children, the DOR is 34 (95% CI, 12–97), in pregnant women it is 165 (95% CI, 73–372), and in the elderly it is 108 (95% CI, 10–1165). Although the authors did not translate the DORs into sensitivity/specificity pairs, they did offer a calculation of how persuasive a positive test and a negative test would be. In children, the prevalence of infections was estimated to be 20% based on the pooled data. A positive test for nitrites would raise this probability to 61% and a negative test would lower the probability to 12%. This is a good result, but not as much as you might hope for. The test appears to be more impressive in pregnant women and the elderly. In pregnant women, a pooled prevalence of infection is 6%. A positive test would raise this probability to 55% and a negative test would lower it to 3%. Among the elderly, where a pooled prevalence rate was estimated at 30%, a positive test would raise the probability to 88% and a negative test would lower it to 11%.

5.5.5 Practical significance in a meta-analysis: What to look for

Do not just look at the statistical significance of a combined estimate in a meta-analysis. Ask yourself if the difference is large enough to have a practical impact. Is it an outcome that patients care about? Is it expressed in units that you can easily interpret?

5.6   Counterpoint: Meta-analysis is overrated

Although most proponents of evidence-based medicine place systematic reviews at the top of the research hierarchy,[3] there are a large number of dissenting voices (Boden 1992; Shapiro 1994; Feinstein 1995). Even strong proponents of meta-analysis have expressed some reservations (Chalmers 1991). The criticisms have come, for the most part, from the earlier years of meta-analysis. The strong criticisms have quieted somewhat recently, but the cautions raised still remain important.

A big problem back then (and something you should still look for) was that the people doing the meta-analyses were statisticians. Now, I like statisticians and think they are very intelligent people, but they do not always have an appreciation of the subtleties of medical practice. A good meta-analysis should have one or more medical experts in charge, because these are the people who can make the best decisions about what studies to use and how to combine them. The medical experts should also have an expert in Statistics on their team, of course, because some of the subtleties of analysis may be missed by the medical specialists.

The selection of studies to include in a meta-analysis is difficult and the process often unintentionally leaves some studies on the outside. This places meta-analysis squarely among the non-randomized studies. You should probably consider the selection of studies in a meta-analysis to represent a convenience sample.[4] This would make meta-analysis a weaker form of evidence than a randomized study.

Another major criticism of meta-analysis is that the technique ends up combining studies that should never be combined. You can think of meta-analysis as a multicenter trial where each center gets to use a different protocol. That's not a good way to do research.

Are these criticisms valid? Does a meta-analysis represent a weaker form of evidence than a randomized clinical trial? Two researchers, in fact, have

---

[3] For example, the hierarchy suggested at the Best Bets website is:

I Strong evidence from at least one published systematic review of multiple well-designed randomized controlled trials

II Strong evidence from at least one published properly designed randomised controlled trial of appropriate size and in an appropriate clinical setting

III Evidence from published well designed trials without randomisation, single group pre-post, cohort, time series or matched case-control studies

IV Evidence from well designed nonexperimental studies from more than one centre or research group

V Opinions of respected authorities, based on clinical evidence, descriptive studies or reports of expert consensus committees. (www.bestbets.org/background/betscats.html).

[4] A convenience sample is a sample where the patients are selected, in part or in whole, at the convenience of the researcher. The researcher makes no attempt, or only a limited attempt, to insure that this sample is an accurate representation of some larger group or population. The classic example of a convenience sample is standing at a shopping mall and selecting shoppers as they walk by to fill out a survey.

done a head-to-head comparison of meta-analysis studies and large scale randomized trials. One group of researchers (LeLorier 1997) found 12 large randomized trials and 19 meta-analyses addressing the same questions. In about one-third of the cases, the results of the two differed, with one suggesting a positive effect of the treatment being studied and the other suggesting no effect. Another group (Cappelleri 1996) selected 61 meta-analyses that included at least one large study. They compared the result of this one study to a meta-analytic summary of the remaining small studies. This research found a smaller degree of discrepancy, and in most of the cases, they found a plausible explanation for this discrepancy.

In summary, meta-analysis, like any other type of research is difficult to do (Berman 2002). And like any other type of research, it has flaws and weaknesses that are unique to its particular methodology. You should not mindlessly trust a research finding just because it has the words 'systematic overview' or 'meta-analysis' in the title.

5.7   Summary—Do the pieces fit together?

There are four factors you should consider when evaluating a systematic review or meta-analysis paper.

Were apples combined with oranges? A review that combines studies that are narrowly drawn offers greater credibility than a combination of heterogenous studies.

Were some apples left on the tree? Look for efforts to ensure that all relevant publications were identified and considered in the meta-analysis.

Were all of the apples rotten? Meta-analysis cannot correct the flaws of the existing research studies and may tend to amplify these flaws.

Did the pile of apples amount to more than just a hill of beans? Look for overall estimates in units that are meaningful and interpretable. Avoid relying on unitless quantities like the effect size.

5.8   On your own

1. Review the following two articles, which include the abstract and some excerpts from the main text. Comment on the degree of heterogeneity found in these studies. Is it serious enough to warrant concern?

Psychiatric diagnoses in 3,275 suicides: a meta-analysis. Arsenault-Lapierre, G., Kim, C., and Turecki, G. *BMC Psychiatry* 2004, 4:37 doi:10.1186/1471-244X-4-37.

Abstract. Background: It is well known that most suicide cases meet criteria for a psychiatric disorder. However, rates of specific disorders vary considerably between studies and little information is known about gender and geographic differences. This study provides overall rates of total and specific psychiatric disorders in suicide completers and presents evidence supporting gender and geographic differences in their relative proportion. **Methods:** We carried out a review of studies in which psychological autopsy studies of suicide completers were performed. Studies were identified by means of MEDLINE database searches and by scanning the reference list of relevant publications. Twenty-three variables were defined, 16 of which evaluating psychiatric disorders. Mantel-Haenszel Weighted Odds Ratios were estimated for these 16 outcome variables. **Results:** Twenty-seven studies comprising 3,275 suicides were included, of which 87.3% (SD 10.0%) had been diagnosed with a mental disorder before their death. There were major gender differences. Diagnoses of substance-related problems (OR = 3.58; 95% CI, 2.78–4.61), personality disorders (OR = 2.01; 95% CI, 1.38–2.95) and childhood disorders (OR = 4.95; 95% CI, 2.69–9.31) were more common among male suicides, whereas affective disorders (OR = 0.66; 95% CI, 0.53–0.83), including depressive disorders (OR = 0.53; 95% CI, 0.42–0.68) were less common among males. Geographical differences are also likely to be present in the relative proportion of psychiatric diagnoses among suicides. **Conclusions:** Although psychopathology clearly mediates suicide risk, gender and geographical differences seem to exist in the relative proportion of the specific psychiatric disorders found among suicide completers.

Excerpt 1. Study identification: To identify studies for this review, the National Library of Medicine (NLM) PubMed database was searched up to December 2002 using English language and human study limits. The Medical Subject Heading (MeSH) terms 'suicide AND psychological autopsy', 'suicide AND psychopathology', 'suicide AND (postmortem diagnoses OR postmortem diagnosis)', and '(mental disorders/*epidemiology) AND prevalence AND ((suicide/*statistics & numerical data) NOT suicide attempts)' were used. Finally, in order to find other articles not obtained through electronic searches, reference lists from original studies as well as from not independent studies were screened.

Study selection: The inclusion criteria for considering articles for this review were as follow. Studies had to: (1) be original, (2) be published in English, (3) contain information on diagnostic distribution, (4) include suicide completers unselected according to specific mental disorders, (5) use of a psychological autopsy method, which for the purpose of this review was considered as the process of reconstructing psychiatric diagnoses based either on interviews with informants (regardless of the specific diagnostic instrument methodology) or on review of multiple official records that contained interviews with informants such as general practitioners, other professionals and relatives or friends, (6) use of standard diagnostic criteria (any versions of the Diagnostic and Statistical Manual of Mental Disorders, the International Classification of Diseases or the Research Diagnostic Criteria).

Studies were excluded if: (1) their sample was not independent from that investigated in another study (see below for criteria on which one was included), (2) they were reports on suicide in one specific diagnostic category, and (3) if diagnoses were simply extracted from medical records without review of multiple sources of information.

A single reviewer (G.A.L.) made a prior screening to identify and select articles. When titles and abstracts were deemed adequate or when they remained too obscure to reach a verdict, full texts were retrieved for further evaluation in conformity with the inclusion and exclusion criteria.

Study assessment: A total of 23 variables were defined, three of which relate to demographic information, four other concern the method of diagnosis, and 16 evaluate the presence of psychiatric diagnoses. To obtain the latter 16 variables, every diagnostic term used in the original studies was categorised into one of the 16 predefined groups. So diagnoses such as 'intermittent depressive disorder' or 'neurotic depression' reported in some studies were coded under 'depressive disorders' variable and diagnoses such as 'alcohol use', 'alcohol misuse', and 'alcohol abuse' were coded as 'alcohol problems'. All substances noted as other than alcohol were coded under 'other substances problems'. These two variables were then recoded as 'any substance problems'. The same was achieved with the 'depressive disorders' and 'bipolar disorders' which were recoded as 'any affective disorders'. Disorders labelled as 'other' or as a subset of various disorders without further specification were left aside. For all studies the most specific diagnosis was considered. That is, when the authors broke down general diagnosis such as 'affective disorder' into 'depressive disorders' and 'bipolar disorders', only these more specific diagnoses were noted and accounted for in our study. When two studies or more were carried on the same population, the study with the largest sample and the most informative report was consistently selected. When multiple diagnoses and principal diagnoses (those deemed by the investigators as more related to the suicide) were reported, preference was given to the former. In four cases, secondary diagnoses were added to principal diagnoses to obtain multiple diagnoses [10–13]. Studies for which controls were selected among psychiatric in-patients or matched to suicides by mental diagnosis, only suicide cases were included in our analysis [12,14]. In the study by Graham and Burvill [15], controls were older suicide completers, and so they were included in our suicide group. In the study by Hawton et al. [10], only diagnoses for suicides obtained by means of an interview were included. In three case-control studies [16–18], not all suicide cases were matched to a control. In these cases, we considered the full suicide sample in the descriptive analyses, but only the control-matched suicides in the quantitative analyses.

Statistical analysis: Descriptive analyses and homogeneity tests were carried out before pooling the data. In order to determine the risks of having had a disorder, suicides and controls were recorded in 2 × 2 tables. These data were then stratified by the 16 outcome variables and Mantel-Haenszel Weighted odds ratios (OR) and 95% confidence intervals (95% CI) were estimated. Gender differences were also explored by means of ORs. Major disorders were then compared between the different demographic areas by means of $\gamma2$ to assess variations in the diagnostic distribution across these demographic areas. All statistical analyses were carried out using Epi Info 6, version 6.04d (CDC, USA; WHO, Geneva, Switzerland).

Excerpt 2. Results: A total of 152 studies were initially identified. After selection according to inclusion/exclusion criteria, 27 studies were included in this review. The most common reasons for exclusion were that (a) no diagnostic distribution was provided ($n = 46$) [6,19–63], (b) samples were pre-selected according to a psychiatric disorder ($n = 30$) [64–93], (c) there was another report on the same sample that either included more subjects or was more informative ($n = 29$) [3,94–121]. Four other studies were about non-completers [122–125]. Another was not in English [126], and others reported only on one type of disorder [127,128], and therefore, they were all excluded. Additional 14 studies [7,129–141] were excluded because the diagnostic criteria were either unspecified or not standard.

The studies by Rich et al. [99] and by Foster et al. [142] were not independent from, respectively, Rich et al. [143] and Foster et al. [144]. Although non-independent, these studies provided information of different quality, and thus, were included in our review. Accordingly, Rich et al. [99] and Foster et al. [142] were considered, respectively in the gender difference analysis and the case-control comparisons, whereas the study by Rich et al. [143] and Foster et al. [144] were considered for the descriptive analysis.

Methodological assessment: Among the 27 studies that were retained, 52% (14/27) were case-control studies. Eighty-one percent (22/27) of the studies were published after 1990. Sixty-seven percent of the studies (18/27) used DSM diagnostic criteria, whereas only 22% (6/27) and 11% (3/27) used the ICD and RDC diagnostic criteria respectively. Multiple diagnoses were investigated in 63% (17/27) of the studies, whereas principal diagnoses only were given for the other 10 studies. A description of the demographic and methodological features of these 27 studies is shown in Table 2.

Demographic features: A total of 3275 suicides were included in our study with a mean number of 121 (standard deviation (SD) 103) suicides per study. There were 11 studies where diagnoses were given by gender for a subtotal of 933 males and 462 females [10,11,18,99,144–150].

There were 14 studies [10–12,14,17,142,145–147,149,151–154] carried out in Europe, including one in Israel [145]. These 14 European studies comprised a total of 1488 suicides. Seven studies were from North America [13,18,143,148,150,155,156] with 794 suicides, three others were from

Australia [15,157,158] with 258 suicides and, finally, three were from Asia [9,16,159]. with 735 suicides.

Diagnostic distribution. The mean percentage of suicides with a psychiatric diagnosis was 87.3% (SD 10.0%). However, only 14 of the 27 studies reported both axes I and II disorders. The remaining 13 studies only assessed axis I diagnoses. The mean percentage of controls with a diagnosis was, as expected, lower (34.9% SD 25.1%). As a comparison, among studies not included because the diagnostic criteria were not specified or not standard, the mean percentage of suicides with a diagnosis was not statistically different from that of the studies included in this review (78.7% SD 21.0%, $\gamma 2 : 2.27, p = 0.13$). On average, 43.2% (SD 18.5%) of suicide cases were diagnosed with any affective disorders (including depressive and bipolar disorders) and 25.7% (SD 14.8%) with other substance problems. In these groups, respectively, depressive disorders and alcohol problems were the most frequent. Finally, personality disorders represented 16.2% (SD 8.6%) of the suicide diagnoses and psychotic disorders, including schizophrenia accounted for 9.2% (SD 10.2%). The samples from the 14 case-control studies were found homogeneous for the 16 outcome variables according to a homogeneity test (results not shown), allowing us to pool the individual studies and determine overall risks. With the exception of organic disorders and adjustment disorders, suicide cases had a higher risk of being diagnosed than controls with each of the diagnoses considered. Of these diagnoses, the risks for psychotic disorders were the highest (OR = 15.38; 95% CI, 3.53–97.82) followed by the variable 'at least one psychiatric disorder' (OR = 10.50; 95% CI, 9.60–13.56). The risk for schizophrenia was also particularly high (OR = 5.56; 95% CI, 3.12–10.24). This is due to the fact that there were only 15 control subjects altogether diagnosed with schizophrenia and two with psychotic disorders. Statistically significant differences were found when male and female suicide cases were compared. However, gender-based comparisons should be considered cautiously as, when available, demographic information indicated that female suicides included in the studies reviewed tended to be older than males. Nevertheless, even considering this potential limitation, the results are interesting. The risks for alcohol (OR = 2.19; 95% CI, 1.63–2.95), other substance problems (OR = 2.02; 95% CI, 1.32–3.10), and any substance problems (OR = 3.58; 95% CI, 2.78–4.61), personality disorders (OR = 2.01; 95% CI, 1.38–2.95) or childhood disorders (OR = 4.95; 95% CI, 2.69–9.31) were greater in male as opposed to female suicides. On the other hand, the risks of having depressive disorders (OR = 0.53; 95% CI, 0.42–0.68) or any affective disorders (OR = 0.66; 95% CI, 0.53–0.83) were lower in males. Analyzing the data according to geographic areas, the diagnostic distribution of the key diagnoses found in suicides differed significantly between world regions, but as mentioned above, potential age-related biases may apply. The American suicides were more often diagnosed with a psychiatric disorder than suicides in the other regions of the world; 89.7 % (SD 4.2 %) of the American suicides had at least one diagnosis, whereas 88.8 % (SD 8.9 %) of the European suicides, 83.0 % (SD 18.4 %) of the Asian suicides and 78.9 % (SD 15.3 %) of the Australian suicides had at least one psychiatric diagnosis.

This is an open source publication. The full free text is available at: www.biomedcentral.com/1471-244X/4/37.

Efficacy of acupuncture for cocaine dependence: a systematic review & meta-analysis. Mills, J.E., Wu, P., Gagnier, J., and Ebbert, J.O. *Harm Reduction Journal* 2005, 2:4 doi:10.1186/1477-7517-2-4.

Abstract. Background: Acupuncture is a commonly used treatment option for the treatment of addictions such as alcohol, nicotine and drug dependence. We systematically reviewed and meta-analyzed the randomized controlled trials of acupuncture for the treatment of cocaine addiction. **Methods:** Two reviewers independently searched 10 databases. Unpublished studies were sought using Clinicaltrials.gov, the UK National Research Register and contacting content experts. Eligible studies enrolled patients with the diagnosis of cocaine dependence of any duration or severity randomly allocated to either acupuncture or sham or other control. We excluded studies of acupuncture methods and trials enrolling patients with polysubstance use or dependence. We abstracted data on study methodology and outcomes. We pooled the studies providing biochemical confirmation of cocaine abstinence. **Results:** Nine studies enrolling 1747 participants met inclusion criteria; 7 provided details for biochemical confirmation of cocaine abstinence. On average, trials lost 50% of enrolled participants (range 0–63%). The pooled odds ratio estimating the effect of acupuncture on cocaine abstinence at the last reported time-point was 0.76 (95% CI, 0.45 to 1.27, P = 0.30, I2 = 30%, Heterogeneity P = 0.19). **Conclusion:** This systematic review and meta-analysis does not support the use of acupuncture for the treatment of cocaine dependence. However, most trials were hampered by large loss to follow up and the strength of the inference is consequently weakened.

Excerpt 1. Methods: Eligible studies enrolled patients with the diagnosis of cocaine dependence of any duration or severity randomly allocated to either acupuncture, sham or other control. Acceptable outcomes measures included: self-reported frequency of cocaine use, self-reported amount of cocaine use, or biochemical confirmation of cocaine abstinence. Biochemical confirmation of cocaine abstinence is defined as the absence of the cocaine metabolite benzoylecognine in the urine. We excluded trials of acupuncture methods and trials enrolling patients with polysubstance use or dependence.

Literature search: Databases searched included: AMED (1985–November 2004), Campbell Collaboration (2001–January 2005), CINAHL (1982–January 2005), Cochrane Library (1998–January 2005), Cochrane

Controlled Trials Registry (January 2005), E-Psyche (1993–January 2005), HTA (1988–January 2005), and MEDLINE (1966–January 2005). We additionally searched the Chinese literature through Wanfang (1997–January 2004) and the Chinese Hospital Knowledge Database (CHKD, 1994–2004). Unpublished studies were also sought using Clinicaltrials.gov and the UK National Research Register. We supplemented this search by hand-searching key journals and searching bibliographies of retrieved trials and reviews. We additionally contacted five authors to identify additional published or unpublished studies and to clarify methodological issues. There were no language restrictions.

Two reviewers (EM, PW) working independently and in duplicate, reviewed the abstracts and full text versions of identified reports and adjudicated their inclusion.

Excerpt 2. Results: The search yielded 83 relevant abstracts. Of these, 20 were retrieved for potential inclusion, four studies were not randomized controlled trials [13–16], four studies investigated methodological issues in acupuncture trials [17–20], two included polysubstance abusers[13,21] and one investigated pharmacothearapy [22]. Chance-adjusted inter-rater agreement was high ($\kappa = 0.96$, 95% CI, 0.91–1) [23–31].

Study characteristics: The nine RCTs were conducted in the USA and included 1747 participants: 488 participants in active groups and 821 assigned to control groups (one RCT did not describe group sizes[25]).

One RCT included only crack cocaine users [27], five RCTs included samples with mixed forms of cocaine abuse (e.g. intravenous, inhaled, or intranasal) and three RCTs did not describe the type of cocaine or the route of administration[26,29,31]. RCTs enrolled participants with different rates of anti-craving medication use and three RCTs included only patients using methadone in addition to cocaine[23,26,31]. Three RCTs enrolled some patients using methadone [24,27,28], 2 RCTs excluded patients who used methadone [25,29] and one did not report the use of anti-craving medication among enrolled subjects [30].

All nine trials employed auricular acupuncture, four employed a specific auricular acupuncture regimen (National Acupuncture Detoxification Association: NADA) and two used a combination of auricular and body points. Five trials had more than one control group [24–26,28,31]or randomized subjects to receive methods including relaxation [26,28,31], anti-craving medication and brainwave modification [24], or psychosocial treatment [25].

Eight trials used urine assays for cocaine metabolites (benzoylecgonine) for biochemical confirmation of abstinence at follow-up; we were able to obtain results from seven of them. Eight trials examined the likelihood of retaining patient participation in the trial, and five trials examined cocaine cravings; no trials reported participant follow-up or relapse.

This is an open source publication. The full free text is available at: www.harmreductionjournal.com/content/2/1/4.

2. Comment on the quality of the search strategy in each of the papers listed above.
3. Comment on the quality of the research studies themselves and on the quality of the studies that were excluded in the two meta-analyses listed above.
4. The forest plot (Figure 5.7) appears in the following article.

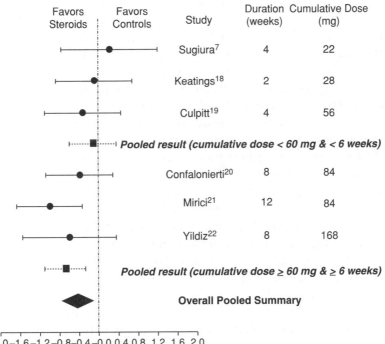

Figure 5.7 Forest plot. This image is from an open source publication. You can find the original article at www.biomedcentral.com/1471-2466/5/3 and this particular figure at www.biomedcentral.com/1471-2466/5/3/figure/F2.

Effects of inhaled corticosteroids on sputum cell counts in stable chronic obstructive pulmonary disease: a systematic review and a meta-analysis. Gan W. Q., SF Paul Man, S. F. P., and Sin, D. D. *BMC Pulmonary Medicine* 2005, 5:3 doi:10.1186/1471-2466-5-3.

Abstract. Background: Whether inhaled corticosteroids suppress airway inflammation in chronic obstructive pulmonary disease (COPD) remains controversial. We sought to determine the effects of inhaled corticosteroids on sputum indices of inflammation in stable COPD. **Methods:** We searched MEDLINE, EMBASE, CINAHL, and the Cochrane Databases for randomized, controlled clinical trials that used induced sputum to evaluate the effect of inhaled corticosteroids in stable COPD. For each chosen study, we calculated the mean differences in the concentrations of sputum cells before and after treatment in both intervention and control groups. These values were then converted into standardized mean differences to accommodate the differences in patient selection, clinical treatment, and biochemical procedures that were employed across original studies. If significant heterogeneity was present ($p < 0.10$), then a random effects model was used to pool the original data. In the absence of significant heterogeneity, a fixed effects model was used. **Results:** We identified six original studies that met the inclusion criteria ($n = 162$ participants). In studies with higher cumulative dose (= 60 mg) or longer duration of therapy (= 6 weeks), inhaled corticosteroids were uniformly effective in reducing the total cell, neutrophil, and lymphocyte counts. In contrast, studies with lower cumulative dose (<60 mg) or shorter duration of therapy (<6 weeks) did not demonstrate a favorable effect of inhaled corticosteroids on these sputum indices. **Conclusions:** Our study suggests that prolonged therapy with inhaled corticosteroids is effective in reducing airway inflammation in stable COPD.

Excerpt: After treatment with inhaled corticosteroids, the total cell counts decreased. Overall, the standardized mean difference between steroid and control groups was −0.43 units (95% confidence interval, CI, −0.75 to −0.11), indicating that inhaled corticosteroids had a favorable effect in reducing total count compared with controls (test for heterogeneity, $p=0.35$). Importantly, the total cumulative dose of inhaled corticosteroids calculated on the basis of mean daily dose and duration of therapy made a material difference to the results. In the studies in which patients were exposed to 60 mg or greater of beclomethasone or its equivalent for the duration of the trial, inhaled corticosteroids were effective in reducing the total sputum cell count (−0.68 units; 95% CI, −1.11 to −0.26). In contrast, trials with cumulative dose of <60 mg did not demonstrate a favorable effect of inhaled corticosteroids on this sputum index (−0.11 units; 95% CI, −0.58 to 0.37). All of the trials with the higher cumulative dose had exposed the trial participants to inhaled corticosteroids for at least 6 weeks; whereas, the trials with the lower cumulative dose was uniformly less than 6 weeks in duration.

This is an open source publication. The full free text is available at: www.biomedcentral.com/1471-2466/5/3.

Interpret this plot and the excerpt from the results section. Comment on the practical impact of this study.

6 What Do All These Numbers Mean?

6.1 Introduction

I have a fictional story that I tell people. It is about someone who comes to my office and says he has trouble understanding a recently published paper. I look at the title: 'In vitro and in vivo assessment of Endothelin as a biomarker of iatrogenically induced alveolar hypoxia in neonates' and say that I understand why he would have trouble with a paper like this. 'Yeah', he says in return, 'I don't understand what this boxplot is on page 3.'

You have already mastered the complex language of medicine, so do not be intimidated by technical statistical terms. I will try to provide some simple explanations of medical terms like confidence interval (CI) and odds ratio (OR), but it is impossible to list all the possible statistical jargon.

When you do come across a statistical term that you are unfamiliar with, do not panic. Here is some general guidance:

1. **Some of the statistical details are there only for the benefit of those who want to reproduce the research.** Most of you recognize that you can safely skim over phrases like 'reverse ion phase chromatography' so you likewise skim over phrases like 'bootstrap confidence intervals using bias corrected percentiles' (Efron 1982). When a statistical method is followed by a reference as in the example above, then you can take some solace in the fact that the authors do not expect you to be familiar with this method.
2. **If a statistical term has several words, focus first on the one word in the term that is most familiar (most often the noun).** You may not know what 'reverse ion phase chromatography' is, but you probably have a good general idea about 'chromatography'. Similarly, with the phrase 'bootstrap confidence intervals using bias corrected percentiles' focus on the term 'confidence intervals'.

You do have to know some statistical terminology, of course. Anyone reading research papers should be familiar with Type I and II errors, odds ratios, survival curves, etc. *A basic appreciation of simple statistical methods is enough for nine out of ten papers.*

6.2 Samples and populations

A population is a collection of items of interest in research. The population represents a group to which you wish to generalize your research. Populations are often defined in terms of *demography, geography, occupation, time, care requirements, diagnosis, or some combination of the above*. In most cases, researchers will not explicitly specify a population, but you can usually infer a reasonable population from the context of the research.

A sample is a subset of a population. A random sample is a subset where every item in the population has the same probability of being in the sample. *Usually, the size of the sample is much less than the size of the population.* The primary goal of much research is to use information collected from a sample to try to characterize a certain population. As such, you should pay a lot of attention to *how representative the sample is of the population.* If there are problems, representatively, consider redefining your population a bit more narrowly. For example, a sample of 85 teenage smokers who volunteer for a research study for a new smoking cessation program might not be considered representative of the population of all teenage smokers, because the participants selected themselves. The sample might be more representative, however, if we restrict our population to those teenage smokers who want to quit.

Example: In a study of vertebral and nonvertebral fracture (Adachi 2002), the researchers selected a sample of '2009 postmenopausal women 50 years and older who were seen in consultation at our tertiary care, university teaching hospital-affiliated office [for a bone fracture] and who were registered in the Canadian Database of Osteoporosis and Osteopenia (CANDOO) patients'. The population that these researchers wished to generalize to would be all postmenopausal women 50 years or older with a bone fracture who live in North America. If you are worried that this would be too difficult to generalize to, you could restrict the population to fractures serious enough to warrant a visit to a tertiary care center.

Example: In a study of post-myocardial infarction pharmacological management in older patients (Di Cecco 2002), a 'comprehensive chart audit was conducted of 142 men and 81 women older than 60 years in an academic primary care practice'. The population that these researchers wanted to generalize to was all post-myocardial patients older than 60 years. Perhaps you might want to restrict the population to men and women who routinely seek out care from a primary care practice.

6.3 Type I and II errors

In many studies, you are interested in choosing between two competing hypotheses. Ideally, you specify the two competing hypotheses before any data collection. You should also specify a decision rule before collecting your data. The decision rule uses information from your sample of data to select one or the other of the two competing hypotheses.

The first hypothesis, often called the null hypothesis or denoted by the symbol H_0, is traditionally a hypothesis that represents the status quo. The null hypothesis is usually reserved for claims of no effect, no association, or no relationship. If you are comparing a new drug to a standard drug, the null hypothesis might be that the average effects of the two drugs are equal.

The second hypothesis, often called the alternative hypothesis and denoted by the symbol H_1 or H_a, represents a claim involving some type of effect or some type of association or relationship. For the study evaluating a new drug, the alternative hypothesis might be that the average effect of the new drug is different than the standard drug (maybe better, maybe worse).

In some situations, your alternative hypothesis may only consider a single direction. For example, if you are comparing a new drug to placebo, the hypothesis that the new drug is worse than placebo is rather uninteresting. It would effectively be no different than if you concluded that the new drug was equivalent to placebo. For these situations, the alternative hypothesis would ignore the possibility of being worse and would restrict itself to the possibility that the new drug is better than placebo.

Hypothesis testing has the danger of oversimplifying the research. Why do you have to choose only between two hypotheses? Why not three or four competing hypotheses? Also, the null hypothesis is perhaps a bit unrealistic. No two drugs are going to have exactly the same level of effectiveness. Would it not be more interesting to look at a null hypothesis that stated that the average effects of the two drugs are close enough to each other that you can feel comfortable using either one? Finally, why do we have to choose? Why can't we just state how much the data changes our degree of belief in the two competing hypotheses?

These types of modifications can be incorporated into hypothesis testing, but too often researchers do not seriously consider modifying the hypotheses but just do things the same old way.

When you are using a decision rule to decide between these two hypothesis, you have to allow for the possibility of error. After all, the decision rule uses information from a sample, which even under the best of circumstances is an imperfect representation of a population. There are actually two types of errors that you can make when choosing between a null and alternative hypothesis.

- A Type I error is *rejecting the null hypothesis when the null hypothesis is true.*
- A Type II error is *accepting the null hypothesis when the null hypothesis is false.*

Consider a new drug that we will put on the market if we can show that it is better than a placebo.

- A Type I error would be *allowing an ineffective drug onto the market.*
- A Type II error would be *keeping an effective drug off the market.*

Both errors are serious, but you should consider the relative importance of each type of error. If your drug is treating a fatal condition, and there is no other effective drug on the market, then a Type II error is very serious because patients without any other hope are being denied an effective treatment. If your drug is treating a less serious condition and is competing against a wide range of drugs already on the market, then from the patient's perspective, a Type II error is less serious. From your company's perspective, a Type II error is still serious because you are being denied the opportunity to compete in a lucrative marketplace.

Statisticians are unique among all of the professions because we admit freely that we make errors. We hope that the probability of these errors is small, and in most situations, we can actually estimate these probabilities. Alpha is defined as the probability of making a Type I error, and beta is defined as the probability of making a Type II error. The complementary probabilities also have names. The confidence level is defined as 1–alpha, and the power is defined as 1–beta.

For a given sample size, there is a trade-off between alpha and beta, not unlike the trade-off between sensitivity and specificity of a diagnostic test. Almost every researcher sets up their decision rule so that alpha, the probability of a Type I error is 0.05. Very few researchers make an attempt to justify this level, and this is a major shortcoming. What they should do is to try to balance alpha and beta according to the costs and severity associated with each type of error. If the cost of a Type I error is trivial and the cost of a Type II error is serious, perhaps the researcher should allow the value of alpha to increase to 0.10 or maybe even higher, so as to ensure that beta, the probability of a Type II error, remains small.

The best way to ensure that both alpha and beta are small is to increase your sample size. A larger sample will typically reduce the probabilities of both types of errors.

Beta (and power) are a bit more difficult to calculate than alpha because you have to specify not only that the null hypothesis is false, but by how much. Typically, you would want to make sure that beta was small for clinically important changes, but you would not worry so much about beta for changes that are clinically trivial. In fact, if your research sample size is so large that beta is miniscule even for clinically trivial changes, then perhaps your sample size is too large. Conversely, if beta is large, even for changes that are clinically important, then you should consider increasing your sample size.

There are extensive formulas and programs that do this sort of calculation. This is often called a power calculation, because the probabilities when the null hypothesis is false are usually stated as power rather than beta.

There are both ethical and economic considerations at work here. A sample size that is too small represents a waste of money, because there is too much of a chance of concluding that the new treatment is equivalent to a placebo, even when it is capable of producing clinically important effects. This ends up wasting time and money, but more importantly, it is an abuse of the goodwill of your research volunteers. People volunteer for a research study for a variety of reasons, but one of the most important is that they want to help out future patients who have the same disease. They are hoping to contribute to the advancement of knowledge, but you have placed them in a research study that has little chance of doing so.

Similarly, a sample size that is too large represents a waste of money and resources, and also raises ethical concerns. There are inconveniences, discomforts, and hazards associated with research, and you should not ask more people to endure these hardships than is needed to demonstrate a clinically important change.

6.4   Confidence interval

We statisticians have a habit of hedging our bets. We always insert qualifiers into our reports, warn about all sorts of assumptions, and never admit to anything more extreme than probable. There is a famous saying: 'Statistics means never having to say you're certain.'

We qualify our statements, of course, because we are always dealing with imperfect information. In particular, we are often asked to make statements about a population (a large group of subjects) using information from a sample (a small, but carefully selected subset of this population). No matter how carefully this sample is selected to be a fair and unbiased representation of the population, relying on information from a sample will always lead to some level of uncertainty.

A confidence interval is a range of values that tries to quantify this uncertainty. Consider it as a range of plausible values. A narrow confidence interval implies high precision; we can specify plausible values to within a tiny range. A wide interval implies poor precision; we can only specify plausible values to a broad and uninformative range.

Consider a recent study of homoeopathic treatment of pain and swelling after oral surgery (Lokken 1995). When examining swelling three days after the operation, they showed that homoeopathy led to 1 mm less swelling on average. The 95% confidence interval (CI), however, ranged from −5.5 to 7.5 mm. From what little I know about oral surgery, this appears to be a very wide interval. This interval implies that neither a large improvement due to homoeopathy nor a large decrement could be ruled out.

Generally, when a CI is very wide like this one, it is an indication of an inadequate sample size, an issue that the authors mention in the discussion section of this chapter.

When you see a CI in a published medical report, you should look for two things. First, does the interval contain a value that implies no change or no effect? For example, with a CI for a difference, look to see whether that interval includes zero. With a CI for a ratio, look to see whether that interval contains one.

Here is an example of a CI that contains the null value. The interval shown below implies no statistically significant change.

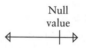

Here is another example of a CI that excludes the null value. If we assume that larger implies better, then the interval shown below would imply a statistically significant improvement.

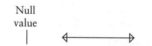

Here is a different example of a CI that excludes the null value. The interval shown below implies a statistically significant decline.

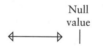

You should also see whether the confidence interval lies partly or entirely within a range of clinical indifference. Clinical indifference represents values of such a trivial size that you would not want to change your current practice. For example, you would not recommend a special diet that showed a one year weight loss of only five pounds. You would not order a diagnostic test that had a predictive value of less than 50%.

Clinical indifference is a medical judgment, and not a statistical judgment. It depends on your knowledge of the range of possible treatments, their costs, and their side effects. As statistician, I can only speculate on what a range of clinical indifference is. I do want to emphasize, however, that if a CI is contained entirely within your range of clinical indifference, then you have clear and convincing evidence to keep doing things the same way (see below).

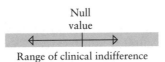

Range of clinical indifference

On the other hand, if part of the confidence interval lies outside the range of clinical indifference, then you should consider the possibility that the sample size is too small (see below).

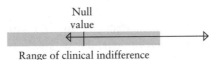

Range of clinical indifference

Some studies have sample sizes that are so large that even trivial differences are declared statistically significant. If your CI excludes the null value but still lies entirely within the range of clinical indifference, then you have a result with statistical significance, but no practical significance (see below).

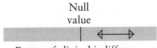
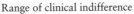

Range of clinical indifference

Finally, if your CI excludes the null value and lies outside the range of clinical indifference, then you have both statistical and practical significance (see below).

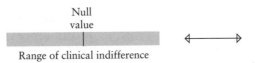

Range of clinical indifference

Example: In a study of trends in hospital admission for lower respiratory illness (Bjor 2003), the annual rate of increase was 3.8% (95% CI, 1.3–6.3) in boys under one year of age and 5.0% (95% CI, 2.4–7.6) in girls under one year of age. Since both of these CIs exclude the value of 0%, you can conclude that there is a statistically significant increase in admission rates. If you presume that a shift of 0.5% or greater in either direction is clinically important, then both of these CIs demonstrate a practical impact.

Example: In a systematic overview of isoflavones or soy phyto-estrogens on serum lipid levels (Yeung 2003), the isoflavones had an insignificant effect on serum total cholesterol showing only a 0.01 mmol/l decline (95% CI, −0.17–0.18). The results were equally disappointing for low density lipoproten (0.00 mmol/l decline, 95% CI, −0.14–0.15), high density lipoprotein (0.01 mmol/l decline, 95% CI, −0.05–0.06), and triglycerides (0.03 mmol/l decline, 95% CI, −0.06–0.12). Since all of these CIs include zero, there is no statistically significant change in these levels. Furthermore, these intervals are so narrow that they would easily be included in any reasonable range of clinical indifference. That makes these findings a definitive negative result.

6.5 *p*-value

A *p*-value is a measure of evidence. A small *p*-value indicates lots of evidence against the null hypothesis. How small is small? Sometimes, researchers will use a stricter cut-off (e.g. 0.01) or a more liberal cut-off (e.g. 0.10). Unfortunately, most researchers give little thought to the cut-off and reflexively use the traditional 0.05 level. As mentioned above, you should set the cut-off depending on how serious a Type I error is compared to a Type II error.

A small *p*-value by itself only tells you half the story because it gives you no information about the magnitude of the change seen. Is there a clinically important difference, or is it trivial? A confidence interval complements the *p*-value well (and some argue that it should even replace the *p*-value) because it provides information about whether the difference seen in this research is clinically important or clinically trivial.

A large *p*-value by itself also tells only half the story. There is little or no evidence against the null hypothesis, but that does not always translate into lots of evidence in favor of the alternative hypothesis. Perhaps your sample size is so small that you do not have much evidence for any particular hypothesis. Again, a confidence interval is more helpful, because a narrow interval (one that fits entirely inside the range of clinical indifference) is strong evidence that nothing important is going on here.

Example: In a study of reviewers of abstracts for a primary care research conference (Montgomery 2002), reviewers rated the abstract on seven categories, with a rating of 1 representing a poor level and 4 representing an excellent level. So the total score ranged from 4 to 28 points. The accepted abstracts had an average rating of 17.4 and the rejected abstracts had a rating of 14.6. The *p*-value for comparing the average rating between the two groups was 0.0003, which is very small. This indicates that you should reject the null hypothesis that the average rating is the same for both groups. The *p*-value, by itself, does not quantify the magnitude of the change, so the authors also included a confidence interval. The 95% confidence interval for the difference in average ratings was 1.3–4.1. You can conclude based on the CI that the difference in average scores is greater than 1 unit, even after allowing for sampling error.

6.6   Odds ratio and relative risk

Both the odds ratio (OR) and the relative risk (RR) compare the likelihood of an event between two groups. Consider the following data on survival of passengers on the *Titanic*. There were 462 female passengers: 308 survived and 154 died. There were 851 male passengers: 142 survived and 709 died (see Table 6.1).

If you saw the movie, Leonardo DiCaprio was one of the 709 male fatalities, and Kate Winslet was one of the 308 female survivors.

Clearly, a male passenger on the *Titanic* was more likely to die than a female passenger. But how much more likely? You can compute the OR or the RR to answer this question.

The OR compares the relative odds of death in each group. For females, the odds were exactly 2–1 against dying (154/308=0.5). For males, the odds were almost 5–1 in favor of death (709/142 = 4.993). The odds ratio is 9.986 (4.993/0.5). There is a tenfold greater odds of death for males than for females.

The RR (sometimes called the risk ratio) compares the probability of death in each group rather than the odds. For females, the probability of death is 33% (154/462 = 0.3333). For males, the probability is 83% (709/851 = 0.8331). The RR of death is 2.5 (0.8331/0.3333). There is a 2.5 greater probability of death for males than for females.

There is quite a difference. Both measurements show that men were more likely to die. But the OR implies that men are much worse off than the relative risk. Which number is a fairer comparison?

The RR measures events in a way that is *interpretable and consistent with the way people really think*. The OR is a bit trickier, since the only people who seem to understand odds well are people who bet on horse races. The big advantage of the OR is its flexibility. For certain research designs, such as a case-control design, you can compute and interpret an OR easily, but a relative risk would be meaningless. You can also easily adjust an OR for covariates.

Both the OR and the RR are measures of relative change. Many researchers believe that measures of relative change paint an incomplete picture of risk. For example, cigarette smoking has a large effect on lung cancer. The figures

Table 6.1.   Mortality outcomes on the Titanic

	Alive	Dead	Total
Female	308	154	462
Male	142	709	851
Total	450	863	1,313

vary a bit depending on the time frame and how you define smoking, but a reasonable estimate is that patients who smoke are ten times more likely to die from lung cancer than patients who do not smoke. Smoking also has an effect on cardiovascular disease. Patients who smoke are twice as likely to die from a heart attack than patients who do not smoke. This seems to imply that heart attacks are less of a problem than lung cancer, but when you actually tally the number of smokers who die from heart attacks, it ends up being greater than the number who die from lung cancer. That is because lung cancer is a relatively uncommon event among nonsmokers, while heart attacks are more frequent. So a doubling of a common risk has more of a public health impact than a tenfold change in a rarer risk.

In contrast to measures of relative change, which involve computing ratios, researchers are now encouraging the use of measures of absolute change, such as risk difference or the number needed to treat. Absolute change involves the computation of a difference rather than a ratio.

The number needed to treat represents the number of patients you would typically have to treat with a new therapy in order to see one additional success compared to the traditional therapy. A low number, like 3, tells you that you will see a lot of extra successes in a short amount of time if you adopt the new therapy. A high number, like 200, means that you will have to treat a lot of patients with the new therapy before you will even see a handful of extra successes.

You can also compute this quantity for adverse effects, such as side effects. In this case, the quantity is usually called the number needed to harm (NNH). A large number is good, because it means that if you give the new therapy to large number of patients, you will only encounter a few more extra side effects. A small number, of course, means that you will see a lot of extra side effects if you adopt the new therapy.

To compute the NNT or NNH, you need to subtract the rate in the treatment group from the rate in the control group and then invert it (divide the difference into 1).

A recently published article on the flu vaccine showed that among the children who received a placebo, 17.9% later had culture confirmed influenza. In the vaccine group, the rate was only 1.3%. This is a 16.6% absolute difference. When you invert this percentage, you get NNT = 6. This means that for every six kids who get the vaccine, you will see one less case of flu on average.

The study also looked at the rate of side effects. In the vaccine group, 1.9% developed a fever. Only 0.8% of the controls developed a fever. This is an absolute difference of 1.1%. When you invert this percentage, you get NNH = 90. This means that for every 90 kids who get the vaccine, you will see one additional fever on average.

Sometimes the ratio between NNT and NNH can prove informative. For this study,

$$\text{NNH/NNT} = 90 / 6 = 15.$$

This tells you that you should expect to see one additional fever for every fifteen cases of flu prevented.

Although I am not a medical expert, the vaccine looks very promising because you can prevent a lot of flu events and only have to put up with a few additional fevers. In general, it takes medical judgment to assess the trade-offs between the benefits of a treatment and its side effects. The NNT and NNH calculations allow you to assess these trade-offs.

6.7 Correlation

A correlation is a measure of the degree of association between two variables.

The correlation coefficient is always between -1 and $+1$. The closer the correlation is to ± 1, the closer to a perfect linear relationship. Here is how I tend to interpret correlations.

- -1.0 to -0.7 strong negative association.
- -0.7 to -0.3 weak negative association.
- -0.3 to $+0.3$ little or no association.
- $+0.3$ to $+0.7$ weak positive association.
- $+0.7$ to $+1.0$ strong positive association.

It is not a perfect rule, and I might stretch the limits a bit depending on the particular problem at hand.

Here is an example. A data-set included in the Data and Story Library (lib.stat.cmu.edu/DASL) measures the 1960 crime rates for 47 states along with a variety of demographic factors. The causes of crime are complex and you cannot draw any valid inferences based on the few graphs presented below. Nevertheless, these graphs illustrate the concept of strong and weak correlation. For example, there is an (almost) strong relationship between police budgets and crime levels. States with more crime have to spend more on police protection (see Figures 6.1–6.3).

There is a weak relationship between education level and crime. States with higher average levels of education do tend to have more crime, but the relationship is more uncertain here.

Finally, there is little or no relationship between unemployment rate and crime.

You should always be cautious about correlations because a large correlation between two variables does not mean that the first variable is the cause of the second. Perhaps it is the second variable that causes the first instead. Someone looking at the first graph (Figure 6.1) might conclude that spending less money on police protection would lead to a lower crime rate.

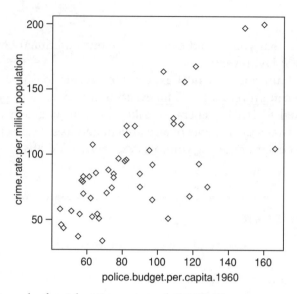

Figure 6.1. Example of an (almost) strong correlation (0.69).

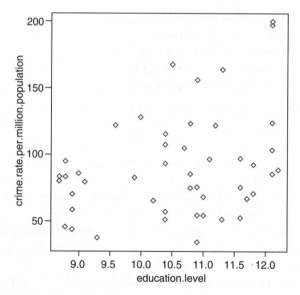

Figure 6.2. Example of a weak correlation (0.32).

That is similar to the story of the statistician who was reviewing records of a fire department and noticed that the more fire engines you sent to the site of a fire, the more damage they caused.

Another problem with a correlation is that it does not take into account additional factors that might represent the underlying cause of the relationship. For example, a study of life expectancies in 40 different countries

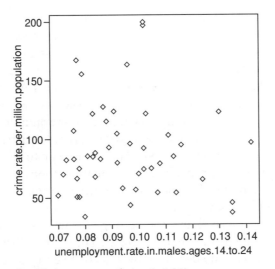

Figure 6.3. Example of little or no correlation (−0.05).

(Rossman 1994) noted a strong relationship between life expectancy and the number of television sets per capita. The surprising relationship was that more television sets were associated with longer lives. It turns out that both availability of consumer goods like televisions and a country's life expectancy were related to a third variable, the wealth of that country. Countries that could afford to buy lots of television sets could also afford to buy adequate health care for their people.

Another example of a misleading correlation appears in a study of patients with Parkinson's disease (Cosentino 2005). The researchers noted a positive association between a particular medication, Levodopa, and the number of times that the patients visited their doctor over the past year. This association, they noted, could be explained by the fact that patients using alternate drugs or using Levodopa in combination with alternate drugs or using alternate drugs alone tended to be much younger.

6.8 Survival curves

Survival data models provide interpretation of data representing the time until an event occurs. In many situations, the event is death, but it can also represent the time to other bad events such as cancer relapse or failure of a medical device. It can also be used to denote time to positive events such as pregnancy.

Survival data models also incorporate one of the complexities of 'time to event' data, the fact that not all patients experience the event during the time frame of the study. So, if we are doing a five-year mortality study, we have the problem of those stubborn patients who refuse to die during the study period. Other patients may move out of town halfway through the study and are lost to follow-up. In a study of medical devices, sometimes the device continues to work up to a certain time, but then has to be removed, not because the device failed, but because the patient got healthier and no longer needed the device.

These observations are called censored observations. With censored observations, the actual time of the event is unknown but we do know that it would not be any earlier than the time that the last evaluation or follow-up visit was done. These censored observations provide partial information. They influence our estimates of survival probability up to the last evaluation or follow-up, but do not provide any information about survival probabilities beyond that point. To disregard this information is dangerous and could seriously bias your results.

Table 6.2 shows survival time for a group of fruit flies and is a subset of a larger data-set found on the Chance website. There are 25 flies in the sample, so the survival probability decreases by 4% (1/25) every time a fly dies.

You have to make some common sense adjustments for ties in the data (when four flies all die on the 47th day, the survival probability declines by 16% not 4%) but otherwise the probabilities are quite easy to compute. Figure 6.4 shows these probabilities over time.

By tradition and for some rather technical reasons, you should use a stair step pattern rather than a diagonal line to connect adjacent survival probabilities, But this does not seriously change the pattern shown.

Now let us alter the experiment. Suppose that totally by accident, a technician leaves the screen cover open on day 70 and all the flies escape. This includes the poor fly that was going to die on the afternoon of the 70th day anyway. You might be tempted to scrap the whole experiment, but really what you have is pretty complete information on survival of the fruit flies up to their 70th day of life. Table 6.3 shows how you would present the data and estimate the survival probabilities.

We clearly have enough data to make several important statements about survival probability. For example, the median survival time is 62 days because roughly half of the flies had died before this day.

Table 6.2. Survival times and estimated survival probabilities for 25 fruit flies.

Days	37	40	44	47	47
Survival probability:	96%	92%	88%	84%	80%
Days	47	47	54	58	58
Survival probability:	76%	72%	68%	64%	60%
Days	59	61	62	62	68
Survival probability:	56%	52%	48%	44%	40%
Days	70	71	72	75	75
Survival probability:	36%	32%	28%	24%	20%
Days	75	79	89	96	96
Survival probability:	16%	12%	8%	4%	0%

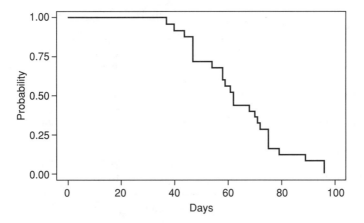

Figure 6.4   A graph of the survival probablities for the data in Table 6.2.

Figure 6.5 shows the survival probabilities of the second experiment. The plus sign on the graph at day 70 is an indication of censored data by the software that drew this graph (SPSS version 13). This graph is identical to the graph in the first experiment up to day 70 after which you can no longer estimate survival probabilities.

By the way, you might be tempted to ignore the ten flies that escaped. But that would seriously bias your results. All of these flies were survivors that lived well beyond the median day of death. If you pretended that they did not exist, you would seriously underestimate the survival probabilities. The median survival time, for example, of the 15 flies that did not escape is only 54 days which is much smaller than the actual median.

Let us look at a third experiment, where the screen cover is left open and all but four of the remaining flies escape. It turns out that those four remaining flies that did not bug out will allow us to still get reasonable estimates of survival probabilities beyond 70 days. Table 6.4 shows the data and the survival probabilities.

Table 6.3.   Survival times and estimated survival probabilities for the same experiment but with the escape of 10 flies on day 70.

Days	37	40	44	47	47
Survival probability:	96%	92%	88%	84%	80%
Days	47	47	54	58	58
Survival probability:	76%	72%	68%	64%	60%
Days	59	61	62	62	68
Survival probability:	56%	52%	48%	44%	40%
Days	70+	70+	70+	70+	70+
Survival probability:	?	?	?	?	?
Days	70+	70+	70+	70+	70+
Survival probability:	?	?	?	?	?

Table 6.4. Survival times and estimated survival probabilities for the same experiment but with the escape of 6 out of 10 flies on day 70.

Days	37	40	44	47	47
Survival probability:	96%	92%	88%	84%	80%
Days	47	47	54	58	58
Survival probability:	76%	72%	68%	64%	60%
Days	59	61	62	62	68
Survival probability:	56%	52%	48%	44%	40%
Days	70+	71	70+	70+	70+
Survival probability:		30%			
Days	75	70+	89	70+	96
Survival probability:	20%		10%		0%

What you need to do is to allocate the remaining 40% survival probability evenly among the four remaining flies. These flies become more important, as each death accounts for a 10% decline in survival probability rather than just a 4% decline at earlier dates.

There is another way of looking at the six flies who escaped. They influence the denominator of the survival probabilities up to day 70 and then totally drop out of the calculations for any further survival probabilities. Because the denominator has been reduced, the jumps at each remaining death are much larger.

Figure 6.6 shows the survival probability estimates from the third experiment.

If you look at the survival probability estimates in the third experiment, they differ only slightly from the survival probabilities in the original experiment. This works out because the mechanism that caused us to lose information on six of the fruit flies was independent of their ultimate survival.

If the censoring mechanism were somehow related to survival prognosis, then you would have the possibility of serious bias in your estimates.

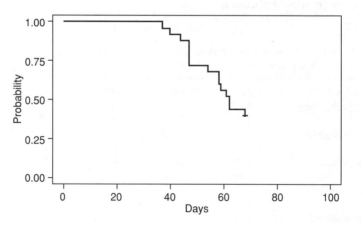

Figure 6.5 A graph of the survival probablities for the data in Table 6.3.

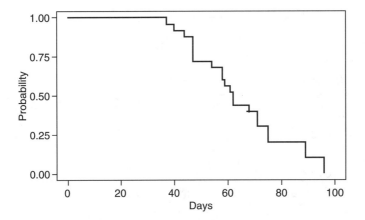

Figure 6.6   A graph of the survival probablities for the data in Table 6.4.

Suppose, for example, that only the toughest of flies (those with the most days left in their short lives) would have been able to escape. Then these censored values would not be randomly interspersed among the remaining survival times, but would constitute some of the larger values. But since these larger values would remain unobserved, you would underestimate survival probabilities beyond the 70th day.

This is known as informative censoring, and it happens more often than you might expect. Suppose someone drops out of a cancer mortality study because they are abandoning the drugs being studied in favor of laetrile treatments down in Mexico. Usually, this is a sign that the current drugs are not working well, so a censored observation here might represent a patient with a poorer prognosis. Excluding these patients would lead to an over-estimate of survival probabilities.

When you see a survival curve in a research paper, there are two ways to interpret it. First, you can get an estimate of the median (or other percent-iles) by projecting horizontally until you intersect with the survival curve and then head down to get your estimate. In the survival curve we have just looked at, you would estimate the median survival as around 65 days (see Figure 6.7).

You can also estimate probabilities for survival at any given time by projecting up from the time and then moving to the left to estimate the probability. In the example below (Figure 6.8), you can see that the 80-day survival probability is approximately 20%.

6.9   Prevalence and incidence

Prevalence and incidence are two measures of how commonly certain diseases are found in a population. They measure two very different

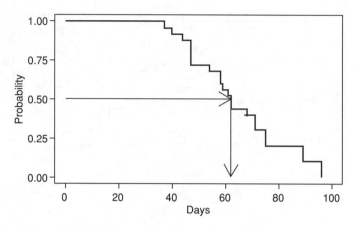

Figure 6.7 Estimating the Median survival time (a bit more than 60 days in this example).

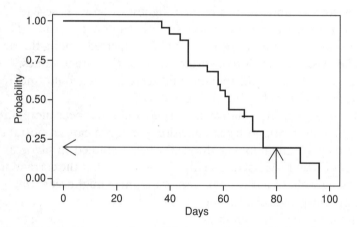

Figure 6.8 Estimating the survival rate (80 day survival is a bit less than 25% in this example).

dimensions of the disease process, but the distinction can sometimes be quite subtle.

Incident cases of disease represent all cases of the diseases that appear during a specific time interval. An example of an incidence would be the number of breast cancer patients newly diagnosed during the past year. Prevalent cases represent the number of cases alive in the population at a specific time point. An example of a prevalence would be all breast cancer patients who are alive during the first day of the current year.

Incidence involves units of time, such as patient-months. For example, in one publication (Smeeth 2004), the incidence of autism is reported as increasing 'from 0.40/10,000 person-years (95% CI 0.30 to 0.54) in 1991 to 2.98/10,000 (95% CI 2.56 to 3.47) in 2001'. By contrast, prevalence is simply a count and is usually expressed as a percentage or as the number of cases per 10,000. Two examples are:

The crude prevalence rates per 1000 of neurological sequelae in twins and singletons after assisted conception and in naturally conceived twins were 8.8, 8.2, and 9.6, and of cerebral palsy 3.2, 2.5, and 4.0, respectively. (Pinborg 2004)

Rheumatoid arthritis (RA)/juvenile rheumatoid arthritis (JRA) was the most frequent diagnosis given. The prevalence rate for JRA in the Oklahoma City Area was estimated as 53 per 100,000 individuals at risk, while in the Billings Area, the estimated prevalence was nearly twice that, at 115 per 100,000. (Mauldin 2004)

These can lead to very different answers, because the probability of finding a case in a given time frame is related to mortality risk. Those patients who have a mild form of disease and survive for a relatively long time have a good chance of being around on the date that you go looking for them. Those patients who die quickly are unlikely to be around on the date that you go looking for them.

Let us consider an example with simulated data (Figure 6.9).

The lines on Figure 6.9 represent the duration of disease with the left end point representing the date that the disease was first diagnosed and the right end point representing the date that the patient died. The line segments are ordered from the time of initial diagnosis with patients diagnosed in 1999 and 2000 at the bottom of the graph and patients diagnosed in 2003 and 2004 at the top of the graph.

Figure 6.10 represents a selection of prevalent cases on the left side, and the darker lines represent those patients who were alive on January 1, 2002.

The right side represents incident cases, and the darker lines represent those patients newly diagnosed with the disease between January 1, 2001 and December 31, 2003.

The prevalent cases include very few patients with short survival time, compared to the incident cases. This becomes more apparent when you reorder the patients by survival time.

In left side of the Figure 6.11, the patients with the shortest survival times appear at the bottom of the graph and the patients with the longest survival

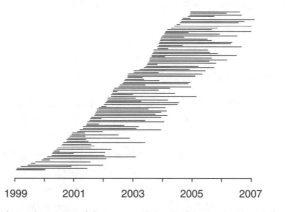

1999   2001   2003   2005   2007

Figure 6.9 Time from diagnosis of disease until death (from a simulated data set).

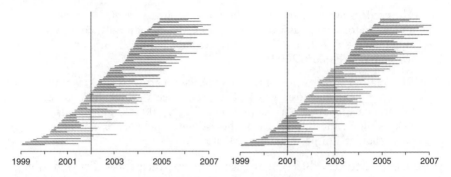

1999   2001   2003   2005   2007   1999   2001   2003   2005   2007

Figure 6.10 Time from diagnosis of disease until death (from a simulated data set). Prevalent cases (cases alive on 1/1/2002) are highlighted on the left and incident cases (cases newly diagnosed between 1/1/2001 and 12/31/2003) are highlighted on the right.

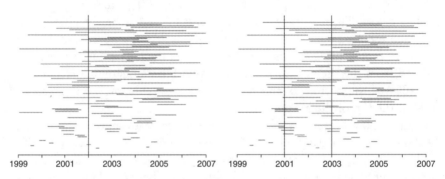

1999   2001   2003   2005   2007   1999   2001   2003   2005   2007

Figure 6.11 Same data as in Figure 6.10 but with values sorted by duration between time of diagnosis and death (most rapidly dying patients appear at the bottom).

times appear at the top. Notice how rarely the patients with short survival times appear among the prevalent cases.

This right hand side of Figure 6.11 shows the incident cases with the patients again sorted by survival time. Notice that the incident cases include a fair number of patients with short survival times.

6.10   On your own

1. Review the following abstracts. Specify what the sample is and define what you think is a reasonable population to which this research is trying to generalize.

The outcome of extubation failure in a community hospital intensive care unit: a cohort study. Seymour, C.W., Martinez, A., Christie, J.D., and Fuchs, B.D. *Critical Care 2004*, 8:R322–R327. **Introduction:** Extubation failure has been associated with poor intensive care unit (ICU) and hospital outcomes in tertiary care medical centers. Given the large proportion of critical care delivered in the community setting, our purpose was to determine the impact of extubation failure on patient outcomes in a community hospital ICU. **Methods:** A retrospective cohort study was performed using data gathered in a 16-bed medical/surgical ICU in a community hospital. During 30 months, all patients with acute respiratory failure admitted to the ICU were included in the source population if they were mechanically ventilated by endotracheal tube for more than 12 hours. Extubation failure was defined as reinstitution of mechanical ventilation within 72 hours ($n = 60$), and the control cohort included patients who were successfully extubated at 72 hours ($n = 93$). **Results:** The primary outcome was total ICU length of stay after the initial extubation. Secondary outcomes were total hospital length of stay after the initial extubation, ICU mortality, hospital mortality, and total hospital cost. Patient groups were similar in terms of age, sex, and severity of illness, as assessed using admission Acute Physiology and Chronic Health Evaluation II score ($p > 0.05$). Both ICU (1.0 vs. 10 days; $p < 0.01$) and hospital length of stay (6.0 vs. 17 days; $p < 0.01$) after initial extubation were significantly longer in re-intubated patients. ICU mortality was significantly higher in patients who failed extubation (odds ratio $= 12.2$, 95% confidence interval [CI] $= 1.5–101$; $p < 0.05$), but there was no significant difference in hospital mortality (odds ratio $= 2.1$, 95% CI $= 0.8–5.4$; $p < 0.15$). Total hospital costs (estimated from direct and indirect charges) were significantly increased by a mean of US\$33,926 (95% CI $=$ US\$22,573–45,280; $p < 0.01$). **Conclusion:** Extubation failure in a community hospital is univariately associated with prolonged inpatient care and significantly increased cost. Corroborating data from tertiary care centers, these adverse outcomes highlight the importance of accurate predictors of extubation outcome.

This is an open source publication. The full free text is available at: ccforum.com/content/8/5/R322.

Effect of paracetamol (acetaminophen) and ibuprofen on body temperature in acute ischemic stroke PISA, a phase II double-blind, randomized, placebo-controlled trial [ISRCTN98608690]. Dippel, D.W.J., van Breda, E.J., van der Worp, H.B., van Gemert, H.M.A., Meijer, R.J., Kappelle, L.J., Koudstaal, P.J., and the PISA-investigators. *BMC Cardiovascular Disorders* 2003, 3:2. **Background:** Body temperature is a strong predictor of outcome in acute stroke. In a previous randomized trial we observed that treatment with high-dose acetaminophen (paracetamol) led to a reduction of body temperature in patients with acute ischemic stroke, even when they had no fever. The purpose of the present trial was to study whether this effect of acetaminophen could be reproduced, and whether ibuprofen would have a similar, or even stronger effect. **Methods:** Seventy-five patients with acute ischemic stroke confined to the anterior circulation were randomized to treatment with either 1,000 mg acetaminophen, 400 mg ibuprofen, or placebo, given 6 times daily during 5 days. Treatment was started within 24 hours from the onset of symptoms. Body temperatures were measured at 2-hour intervals during the first 24 hours, and at 6-hour intervals thereafter. **Results:** No difference in body temperature at 24 hours was observed between the three treatment groups. However, treatment with high-dose acetaminophen resulted in a 0.3°C larger reduction in body temperature from baseline than placebo treatment (95% CI, 0.0–0.6°C). Acetaminophen had no significant effect on body temperature during the subsequent four days compared to placebo, and ibuprofen had no statistically significant effect on body temperature during the entire study period. **Conclusions:** Treatment with a daily dose of 6,000 mg acetaminophen results in a small, but potentially worthwhile decrease in body temperature after acute ischemic stroke, even in normothermic and subfebrile patients. Further, large randomized clinical trials are needed to study whether early reduction of body temperature leads to improved outcome.

This is an open source publication. The full free text is available at: www.biomedcentral.com/1471-2261/3/2.

2. Interpret the CIs reported in the same set of abstracts. Specify a range of clinical indifference as best you can and interpret these intervals with respect to that range.

Elevated white cell count in acute coronary syndromes: relationship to variants in inflammatory and thrombotic genes. Byrne, C.E., Fitzgerald, A., Cannon, C.P., Fitzgerald, D.J., and Shields, D.C. *BMC Medical Genetics* 2004, 5:13. **Background:** Elevated white blood cell counts (WBC) in acute coronary syndromes (ACS) increase the risk of recurrent events, but it is not known if this is exacerbated by pro-inflammatory factors. We sought to identify whether pro-inflammatory genetic variants contributed to alterations in WBC and C-reactive protein (CRP) in an ACS population. **Methods:** WBC and genotype of interleukin 6 (IL-6 G-174C) and of interleukin-1 receptor antagonist (IL1RN intronic repeat polymorphism) were investigated in 732 Caucasian patients with ACS in the OPUS-TIMI-16 trial. Samples for measurement of WBC and inflammatory factors were taken at baseline, i.e. Within 72 hours of an acute myocardial infarction or an unstable angina event. **Results:** An increased white blood cell count (WBC) was associated with an increased C-reactive protein ($r = 0.23$, $p < 0.001$) and there was also a positive correlation between levels of β-fibrinogen and C-reactive protein ($r = 0.42$, $p < 0.0001$). IL1RN and IL6 genotypes had no significant impact upon WBC. The difference in median WBC between the two homozygote IL6 genotypes was $0.21/mm^3$ (95% CI, $-0.41, 0.77$), and $-0.03/mm^3$ (95% CI, $-0.55, 0.86$) for IL1RN. Moreover, the composite endpoint was not significantly affected by an interaction between WBC and the IL1 ($p = 0.61$) or IL6 ($p = 0.48$)

genotype. **Conclusions:** Cytokine pro-inflammatory genetic variants do not influence the increased inflammatory profile of ACS patients.

This is an open source publication. The full free text is available at: www.biomedcentral.com/1471-2350/5/13.

Effect of paper quality on the response rate to a postal survey: a randomised controlled trial. [ISRCTN32032031] Clark, T.J., Khan, K.S., and Gupta, J.K. *BMC Medical Research Methodology* 2001, 1:12. **Background:** Response rates to surveys are declining and this threatens the validity and generalizability of their findings. We wanted to determine whether paper quality influences the response rate to postal surveys **Methods:** A postal questionnaire was sent to all members of the British Society of Gynaecological Endoscopy (BSGE). Recipients were randomized to receiving the questionnaire printed on standard quality paper or high quality paper. **Results:** The response rate for the recipients of high quality paper was 43/195 (22%) and 57/194 (29%) for standard quality paper (relative rate of response 0.75, 95% CI, 0.33–1.05, $p = 0.1$ **Conclusion:** The use of high quality paper did not increase response rates to a questionnaire survey of gynaecologists affiliated to an endoscopic society.

This is an open source publication. The full free text is available at: www.biomedcentral.com/1471-2288/1/12.

Do English and Chinese EQ-5D versions demonstrate measurement equivalence? an exploratory study. Luo, N., Chew, L.H., Fong, K.Y., Koh, D.R., Ng, S.C., Yoon, K.H., Vasoo, S., Li, S.C., and Thumboo, J. *Health and Quality of Life Outcomes* 2003, 1:7. **Background:** Although multiple language versions of health-related quality of life instruments are often used interchangeably in clinical research, the measurement equivalence of these versions (especially using alphabet vs. pictogram-based languages) has rarely been assessed. We therefore investigated the measurement equivalence of English and Chinese versions of the EQ-5D, a widely used utility-based outcome instrument. **Methods:** In a cross-sectional study, either EQ-5D version was administered to consecutive outpatients with rheumatic diseases. Measurement equivalence of EQ-5D item responses and utility and visual analog scale (EQ-VAS) scores between these versions was assessed using multiple regression models (with and without adjusting for potential confounding variables), by comparing the 95% confidence interval (95%CI) of score differences between these versions with predefined equivalence margins. An equivalence margin defined a magnitude of score differences (10% and 5% of entire score ranges for item responses and utility/ EQ-VAS scores, respectively) which was felt to be clinically unimportant. **Results:** Sixty-six subjects completed the English and 48 subjects the Chinese EQ-5D. The 95% CI of the score differences between these versions overlapped with but did not fall completely within pre-defined equivalence margins for 4 EQ-5D items, utility and EQ-VAS scores. For example, the 95%CI of the adjusted score difference between these EQ-5D versions was -0.14 to $+0.03$ points for utility scores and -11.6 to $+3.3$ points for EQ-VAS scores (equivalence margins of −0.05 to +0.05 and −5.0 to +5.0 respectively). **Conclusion:** These data provide promising evidence for the measurement equivalence of English and Chinese EQ-5D versions.

This is an open source publication. The full free text is available at: www.hqlo.com/content/1/1/7.

3. Read the following abstract. The RR for cryotherapy has been removed. Calculate this value using the information provided in the abstract. Interpret this relative risk and the associated CI.

Treatment of retinopathy of prematurity with topical ketorolac tromethamine: a preliminary study. Avila-Vazquez, M., Maffrand, R., Sosa, M., Franco, M., De Alvarez, B.V., Cafferata, M.L., and Bergel, E. *BMC Pediatrics* 2004, 4(1): 15. **Background:** Retinopathy of Prematurity (ROP) is a common retinal neovascular disorder of premature infants. It is of variable severity, usually heals with mild or no sequelae, but may progress to blindness from retinal detachments or severe retinal scar formation. This is a preliminary report of the effectiveness and safety of a new and original use of topical ketorolac in preterm newborn to prevent the progression of ROP to the more severe forms of this disease. **Methods:** From January 2001 to December 2002, all 59 preterm newborns with birthweight less than 1,250 g or gestational age less than 30 weeks of gestational age admitted to neonatal intensive care were eligible for treatment with topical ketorolac (0.25 mg every 8 hours in each eye). The historical comparison group included all 53 preterm newborns, with the same inclusion criteria, admitted between January 1999 and December 2000. **Results:** Groups were comparable in terms of weight distribution, Apgar score at 5 minutes, incidence of sepsis, intraventricular hemorrhage and necrotizing enterocolitis. The duration of oxygen therapy was significantly longer in the control group. In the ketorolac group, among 43 children that were alive at discharge, one (2.3%) developed threshold ROP and cryotherapy was necessary. In the comparison group 35 children survived, and six child (17%) needed cryotherapy (relative risk [**DELETED**], 95% CI, 0.00–0.80, $p = 0.041$). Adjusting by duration of oxygen therapy did not significantly change these results. Adverse effects attributable to ketorolac were not detected. **Conclusions:** This preliminary report suggests that ketorolac in the form of an ophthalmic solution can reduce the risk of developing severe ROP in very preterm newborns, without producing significant adverse side effects. These results, although promising, should be interpreted with caution because of the weakness of the study design. This is an inexpensive and simple intervention that might ameliorate the progression of a disease with devastating consequences for children and their families. We believe that next logical step would be to assess the effectiveness of this intervention in a randomized controlled trial of adequate sample size.

This is an open source publication. The full free text is available at: www.biomedcentral.com/1471-2431/4/15.

4. Read the following abstract. The relative risks for reduced blood loss, shivering, and pyrexia have been removed. Calculate these values using the information provided in the abstract. Interpret these relative risks and their associated CIs.

Misoprostol for treating postpartum haemorrhage: a randomized controlled trial [ISRCTN72263357]. Hofmeyr, G.J., Ferreira, S., Nikodem, V.C., Mangesi, L., Singata, M., Jafta, Z., Maholwana, B., Mlokoti, Z., Walraven, G., and Gulmezoglu, A.M. *BMC Pregnancy & Childbirth* 2004, 4(1): 16. **Background:** Postpartum haemorrhage remains an important cause of maternal death despite treatment with conventional therapy. Uncontrolled studies and one randomized comparison with conventional oxytocics have reported dramatic effects with high-dose misoprostol, usually given rectally, for treatment of postpartum hemorrhage, but this has not been evaluated in a placebo-controlled trial. **Methods:** The study was conducted at East London Hospital Complex, Tembisa and Chris Hani Baragwanath Hospitals, South Africa. Routine active management of the third stage of labor was practiced. Women with more than usual postpartum bleeding thought to be related to inadequate uterine contraction were invited to participate, and to sign informed consent. All routine treatment was given from a special 'Postpartum Haemorrhage Trolley'. In addition, participants who consented were enrolled by drawing the next in a series of randomised treatment packs containing either misoprostol 5 × 200 microg or similar placebo, which were given 1 orally, 2 sublingually and 2 rectally. **Results:** With misoprostol there was a trend to reduced blood loss ≥500 ml in 1 hour after enrolment measured in a flat plastic 'fracture bedpan', the primary outcome (6/117 vs. 11/120, relative risk [DELETED]; 95% confidence interval 0.21–1.46). There was no difference in mean blood loss or haemoglobin level on day 1 after birth < 6 g/dl or blood transfusion. Side effects were increased, namely shivering (63/116 vs. 30/118; [DELETED], 1.50–3.04) and pyrexia > 38.5 degrees C (11/114 vs. 2/118; [DELETED], 1.29–25). In the misoprostol group three women underwent hysterectomy of whom 1 died, and there were two further maternal deaths. **Conclusions:** Because of a lower than expected incidence of the primary outcome in the placebo group, the study was underpowered. We could not confirm the dramatic effect of misoprostol reported in several unblinded studies, but the results do not exclude a clinically important effect. Larger studies are needed to assess substantive outcomes and risks before misoprostol enters routine use.

This is an open source publication. The full free text is available at: www.biomedcentral.com/1471-2393/4/16.

5. Read the following abstract. The authors report an adjusted OR of 5.0 for low socioeconomic index. Compute a crude OR using the data that

appears in the abstract. Does it differ much from the adjusted OR? Interpret the adjusted odds ratio and its associated CI.

Socioeconomic disparities in intimate partner violence against Native American women: a cross-sectional study. Malcoe, L.H., Duran, B.M., and Montgomery, J.M. *BMC Medicine* 2004, 2(1): 20. **Background:** Intimate partner violence (IPV) against women is a global public health problem, yet data on IPV against Native American women are extremely limited. We conducted a cross-sectional study of Native American women to determine prevalence of lifetime and past-year IPV and partner injury; examine IPV in relation to pregnancy; and assess demographic and socioeconomic correlates of past-year IPV. **Methods:** Participants were recruited from a tribally oper-ated clinic serving low-income pregnant and childbearing women in south-west Oklahoma. A self-administered survey was completed by 312 Native American women (96% response rate) attending the clinic from June through August 1997. Lifetime and past-year IPV were measured using modified 18-item Conflict Tactics Scales. A socioeconomic index was created based on partner's education, public assistance receipt, and poverty level. **Results:** More than half (58.7%) of participants reported lifetime physical and/or sexual IPV; 39.1% experienced severe physical IPV; 12.2% reported partner-forced sexual activity; and 40.1% reported lifetime partner-perpet-rated injuries. A total of 273 women had a spouse or boyfriend during the previous 12 months (although all participants were Native American, 59.0% of partners were non-Native). Among these women, past-year preva-lence was 30.1% for physical and/or sexual IPV; 15.8% for severe physical IPV; 3.3% for forced partner-perpetrated sexual activity; and 16.4% for intimate partner injury. Reported IPV prevalence during pregnancy was 9.3%. Pregnancy was not associated with past-year IPV (OR = 0.9). Past-year IPV prevalence was 42.8% among women scoring low on the socio-economic index, compared with 10.1% among the reference group. After adjusting for age, relationship status, and household size, low socioeco-nomic index remained strongly associated with past-year IPV (OR = 5.0; 95% CI, 2.4, 10.7). **Conclusions:** Native American women in our sample experienced exceptionally high rates of lifetime and past-year IPV. Addition-ally, within this low-income sample, there was strong evidence of socio-economic variability in IPV. Further research should determine prevalence of IPV against Native American women from diverse tribes and regions, and examine pathways through which socioeconomic disadvantage may in-crease their IPV risk.

This is an open source publication. The full free text is available at: www.biomedcentral.com/1741-7015/2/20.

6. Read the following abstract. The crude ORs for fissured tongue and for benign migratory glossitis have been removed from this abstract. Calculate

these values using the information provided in the abstract. Interpret these odds ratios and the associated CIs.

Tongue lesions in psoriasis: a controlled study. Daneshpazhooh, M., Moslehi, H., Akhyani, M., and Etesami, M. *BMC Dermatology* 2004: 4(1); 16. **Background:** Our objective was to study tongue lesions and their significance in psoriatic patients. **Methods:** The oral mucosa was examined in 200 psoriatic patients presenting to Razi Hospital in Tehran, Iran, and 200 matched controls. **Results:** Fissured tongue (FT) and benign migratory glossitis (BMG) were the two most frequent findings. FT was seen more frequently in psoriatic patients ($n = 66$, 33%) than the control group ($n = 19$, 9.5%) [OR: [DELETED]; 95% CI, 2.61–8.52] (p-value < 0.0001). BMG, too, was significantly more frequent in psoriatic patients (28 cases, 14%) than the control group (12 cases, 6%) (OR: [DELETED]; 95% CI, 1.20–5.50) (p-value < 0.012). In 11 patients (5.5%), FT and BMG coexisted. FT was more frequent in pustular psoriasis (7 cases, 53.8%) than erythemato-squamous types (56 cases, 30.4%). On the other hand, the frequency of BMG increased with the severity of psoriasis in plaque-type psoriasis assessed by psoriasis area and severity index (PASI) score. **Conclusions:** Nonspecific tongue lesions are frequently observed in psoriasis. Further studies are recommended to substantiate the clinical significance of these seemingly nonspecific findings in suspected psoriatic cases.

This is an open source publication. The full free text is available at: www.biomedcentral.com/1471-5945/4/16.

7. Read the following abstract. The authors report an adjusted OR of 0.19 for presence of contraindication. Compute a crude OR using the data that appears in the abstract. Does it differ much from the adjusted OR? Interpret the adjusted OR and its associated CI.

Breastfeeding practices in a cohort of inner-city women: the role of contraindications. England, L., Brenner, R., Bhaskar, B., Simons-Morton, B., Das, A., Revenis, M., Mehta, N., and Clemens, J. *BMC Public Health* 2003, 3(1): 28. **Background:** Little is known about the role of breastfeeding contraindications in breastfeeding practices. Our objectives were to (1) identify predictors of breastfeeding initiation and duration among a cohort of predominantly low-income, inner-city women, and (2) evaluate the contribution of breastfeeding contraindications to breastfeeding practices. **Methods:** Mother–infant dyads were systematically selected from three District of Columbia hospitals between 1995 and 1996. Breastfeeding contraindications and potential predictors of breastfeeding practices were identified through medical record reviews and interviews conducted after delivery (baseline). Interviews were conducted at 3–7 months postpartum and again at 7–12 months postpartum to determine breastfeeding initiation rates and duration. Multivariable logistic regression analysis was used to identify baseline factors associated with initiation of breastfeeding. Cox proportional hazards models were generated to identify baseline factors associated with duration of breastfeeding. **Results:** Of 393 study participants, 201 (51%) initiated breastfeeding. A total of 61 women (16%) had at lease one documented contraindication to breastfeeding; 94% of these had a history of HIV infection and/or cocaine use. Of the 332 women with no documented contraindications, 58% initiated breastfeeding, vs. 13% of women with a contraindication. In adjusted analysis, factors most strongly associated with breastfeeding initiation were presence of a contraindication (adjusted OR [AOR], 0.19; 95% confidence interval [CI], 0.08–0.47), and mother foreign-born (AOR, 4.90; 95% CI, 2.38–10.10). Twenty-five percent of study participants who did not initiate breastfeeding cited concern about passing dangerous things to their infants through breast milk. Factors associated with discontinuation of breastfeeding (all protective) included mother foreign-born (hazard ratio [HR], 0.55; 95% CI, 0.39–0.77) increasing maternal age (HR for 5-year increments, 0.80; 95% CI, 0.69–0.92), and infant birth weight > or = 2500 grams (HR, 0.45; 95% CI, 0.26–0.80). **Conclusions:** Breastfeeding initiation rates and duration were suboptimal in this inner-city population. Many women who did not breastfeed had contraindications and/or were concerned about passing dangerous things to their infants through breast milk. It is important to consider the prevalence of contraindications to breastfeeding when evaluating breastfeeding practices in high-risk communities.

This is an open source publication. The full free text is available at: www.biomedcentral.com/1471-2458/3/28.

8. Read the following abstract. The number needed to treat (NNT) for 60% of attempts at sexual intercourse being successful, and the number needed to harm (NNH) for treatment-related adverse events have been removed. Calculate these values using the information provided in the abstract. Interpret these values and their associated CIs.

Sildenafil (Viagra) for male erectile dysfunction: a meta-analysis of clinical trial reports. Moore, R.A., Edwards, J.E., and McQuay, H.J. *BMC Urology* 2002, 2(1): 6. **Background:** Evaluation of company clinical trial reports could provide information for meta-analysis at the commercial introduction of a new technology. **Methods:** Clinical trial reports of sildenafil for erectile dysfunction from September 1997 were used for meta-analysis of randomized trials (at least four weeks duration) and using fixed or dose optimization regimens. The main outcome sought was an erection, sufficiently rigid for penetration, followed by successful intercourse, and conducted at home. **Results:** Ten randomized controlled trials fulfilled the inclusion criteria (2,123 men given sildenafil and 1,131 placebo). NNT or NNH were calculated for important efficacy, adverse event and discontinuation outcomes. Dose optimization led to at least 60% of attempts at sexual intercourse being successful in 49% of men, compared with 11% with placebo; the NNT was [DELETED] (95% confidence interval 2.3–3.3). For global improvement in erections the NNT was 1.7 (1.6–1.9). Treatment-related adverse events occurred in 30% of men on dose optimized sildenafil compared with 11% on placebo; the NNH was [DELETED] (4.3–7.3). All cause discontinuations were less frequent with sildenafil (10%) than with placebo (20%). Sildenafil dose optimization gave efficacy equivalent to the highest fixed doses, and adverse events equivalent to the lowest fixed doses. **Conclusion:** This review of clinical trial reports available at the time of licencing agreed with later reviews that had many more trials and patients. Making reports submitted for marketing approval available publicly would provide better information when it was most needed, and would improve evidence-based introduction of new technologies.

This is an open source publication. The full free text is available at: www.biomedcentral.com/1471-2490/2/6.

9. The following Kaplan-Meier survival curve represents survival probabilities for mechanically ventilated patients with severe acute respiratory syndrome (SARS). Estimate the median survival for the subgroup of patients with pneumothorax. Estimate the median survival for the subgroup without pneumothorax. In each subgroup, estimate the fraction of patients who will be expected to survive at least 25 days.

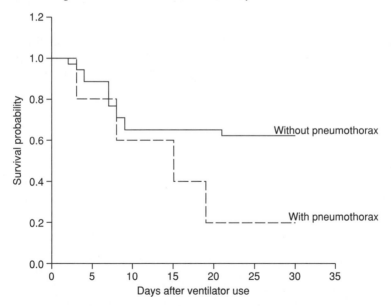

This image is from an open source publication. You can find the original article at: www.ccforum.com/content/9/4/R440 and this particular figure at: www.ccforum.com/content/9/4/r440/figure/F1.

10. The following Kaplan-Meier survival curve represents the probability that a patient avoids readmission after an initial visit to a hospital in

Manchester, UK. For patients in the affluent class, estimate the proportion who were readmitted in the first 200 days. Estimate that same proportion for patients in the deprived class.

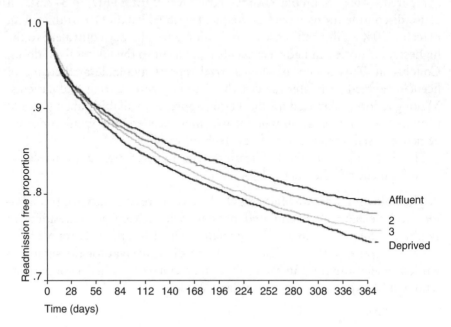

This image is from an open source publication. You can find the original article at: www.biomedcentral.com/1471-227X/5/1 and this particular figure at: www.biomedcentral.com/1471-227x/5/1/figure/F1.

7 Where Is the Evidence? Searching for Information

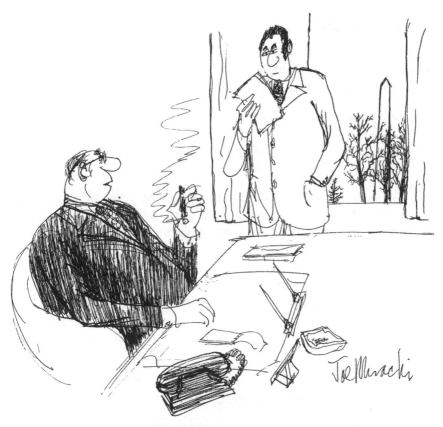

"That's the gist of what I want to say. Now get me some statistics to base it on."

7.1. Introduction

In a book like this, it would be difficult to give a comprehensive overview of how to search the published literature to find all the research studies associated with a particular treatment or a particular disease. You should discuss any serious literature search with a professional librarian.

Here, I want to give you a quick overview of some of the issues associated with searching. I do a lot of searches to find good teaching examples. That is not quite the same thing as finding all the studies associated with a disease, but you may find some of the tricks I have learned to be helpful.

7.2   PICO format

When you are searching for information, it helps to use a structured format for your question. The PICO format works very well. To focus your question well, you should specify:

- P = patient group or problem
- I = intervention
- C = comparison intervention or group
- O = outcome

Not every question fits perfectly into this structure. You may also find that your question does not involve a comparison group.

A question about prenatal smoking and birth weights could easily be fit into the PICO format.

Does the use of smoking cessation programs (I) in women who are pregnant (P) lead to an improvement in birth weight (O) compared to simply offering advice and encouragement about the importance of quitting smoking (C)?

7.3   Search high-level sources first

I was trying to track down an article that I remembered from several years ago. It was an evaluation of smoking cessation programs for pregnant mothers to try to improve the birth outcomes, especially an increase in birth weight.

Normally, it is best to go to high-level sources, such as the Cochrane database, bestbets.org, or guidelines.gov first. There is a very nice Cochrane review, which we will see details about later. The search at bestbets.org was a bust, but guidelines.gov had a nice guideline.

- 'DoD/VA clinical practice guideline for management of uncomplicated pregnancy' www.guidelines.gov/summary/summary.aspx?doc_id=3847 &nbr=3062

It was not quite what I was looking for, but it was still worth reading. This guideline had the following comments about smoking during pregnancy:

I-5 Screening for Tobacco Use—Offer Cessation—Week: 6–8

The Working Group's Recommendations for Women in Low Risk Pregnancy:

1. Strongly recommend routine screening for tobacco use in pregnancy at the initial prenatal visit. For patients who smoke, recommend assessment of smoking status at each subsequent prenatal visit. (Lumley, Oliver, and Waters, 2001; Mullen et al., 1991) (QE: I; Overall Quality: Good; R: A)
2. If the screening is positive, cessation should be strongly recommended. (Wisborg et al., 2000; Panjari et al., 1999; Dolan-Mullen, Ramirez, & Groff, 1994) (QE: I; Overall Quality: Good; R: A)
3. There is insufficient data to recommend for or against pharmacologic therapy for tobacco cessation in pregnancy.

Notice the cryptic notes in parentheses after items 1 and 2. This a grading system on the quality of the evidence, and you have to be sure you understand the codes properly. Some systems use number codes and some use letter codes. Even worse, for some systems, low numbers or letters represent the best quality evidence and for other systems low numbers or letters represent the lowest quality evidence. So you have to read the fine print.

For this particular guideline, QE: I represents 'Evidence obtained from at least one properly randomized controlled trial.' You can also discover that 'Overall Quality: Good' means that the evidence is directly linked to the health outcome, as opposed to an intermediate or surrogate outcome. Finally, the phrase 'R:A' means 'A strong recommendation that the intervention is always indicated and acceptable'.

7.4 Searching in PubMed

For a complex search in PubMed, it can sometimes help break the search into individual pieces and then combine the pieces together. So you should first take a look at how many references you would find if you looked at 'smoking cessation' (10,621 references), and then pregnancy (570,261 references), and then birth weight (29,446 references). All of these numbers are large, which reassures you that you are searching using the right words. In contrast, if you had searched on 'stopping smoking' rather than 'smoking cessation', you would have only found 661 references, which is too small a base when you start combining it with the other terms. Now combine the terms together:

- 'smoking cessation' and 'pregnancy' (697 references)
- 'smoking cessation' and 'birth weight' (73 references)
- 'pregnancy' and 'birth weight' (18,529 references)

The combination of all of these terms produces 69 references. When you still have a large number of references, you then have the luxury of looking for a meta-analysis of these studies to save yourself the effort of reading a bunch of individual studies. You can click on the LIMITS tab in the PubMed search, or you can add the term 'Meta-Analysis [pt]' to your search criteria. This final search yields two meta-analyses:

1. Lumley, J., Oliver, S.S., Chamberlain, C., and Oakley, L. Interventions for promoting smoking cessation during pregnancy. *Cochrane Database Syst Rev.* 2004 Oct 18;(4):CD001055. Review. PMID: 15495004 [PubMed - indexed for MEDLINE]
2. DiFranza, J. R., and Lew, R. A. Effect of maternal cigarette smoking on pregnancy complications and sudden infant death syndrome. *J Fam Pract.* 1995 Apr;40(4):385–94.
   PMID: 7699353 [PubMed - indexed for MEDLINE]

and the first one listed is the one I wanted.

7.4.1   PubMed tags

The '[pt]' is an example of a PubMed tag. These tags allow you to specify exactly what part of the PubMed record you want to search for.

For example, I was searching on Schiavo to see if there were any interesting commentaries about this case in PubMed Central. But when I searched simply on 'Schiavo,' PubMed gave me 10 articles where one of the authors had a last name of Schiavo. I could search instead for 'Schiavo [ti]' which would limit my search to those articles where the word 'Schiavo' appeared in the title of the publication.

Other useful tags in PubMed are:

- [au] author name
- [la] language
- [ta] journal title
- [dp] date of publication

The [ta] tag is very useful when the name of the journal (e.g. Circulation) is also a commonly used medical term. You can also search by the journal's ISSN number if you know it.

The [dp] tag uses the YYYY/MM/DD format and you can specify only the year or only the year/month. You can also specify a range using a colon between the two dates. Finally, you can search the last X days by specifying 'last X days [dp]' in your search. This also works for the last X months and the last X years. The [tiab] tag allows you to search for words in either the title or the abstract.

The 'free full text [sb]' tag will retrieve only those articles with free full text on the web. For example, searching on 'L'Abbe plot' yielded seven references, but when I searched on 'free full text [sb] L'Abbe plot' I got the two articles which had free full text on the web. When you are looking for good teaching examples, it is wonderful to search for publications that you can link to directly, knowing that everyone who reads your pages will be able to view the full article if they so desire.

You can also search for certain publication types such as Review, Clinical Trial, or Editorial using the [pt] tag.

7.4.2 MeSH terms

You could have refined this search using MeSH terms. MeSH terms are especially helpful for a term like 'heart attack' that is too vague from a medical viewpoint. This vagueness causes two problems. First, 'heart' and 'attack' are common words with multiple meanings and uses. These words may appear far separated from each other in an article that is totally unrelated to heart attacks. Second, the words 'heart attack' could describe conditions like 'Myocardial Infarction' or 'Coronary Arteriosclerosis' or 'Coronary Thrombosis' or 'Congestive Heart Failure' and would thus produce too broad a range of conditions.

7.4.3 PubMed filters

Professionals who use PubMed regularly have developed specialized filters that try to accurately identify studies of a particular type. For example, to search for studies of prognosis, you can use the following search terms:

- (incidence[MeSH:noexp] OR mortality[MeSH Terms] OR follow-up studies[MeSH:noexp] OR prognos*[Text Word] OR predict*[Text Word] OR course*[Text Word])

to get a highly sensitive search (a long list that is unlikely to exclude studies in this category) or

- (prognos*[Title/Abstract] OR (first[Title/Abstract] AND episode[Title/Abstract]) OR cohort[Title/Abstract])

to get a highly specific search (a short list that is unlikely to include irrelevant studies).

You can combine these filters with medical terms to make sure that your search focuses on the right type of study. Further details about these filters are at the PubMed website: www.ncbi.nlm.nih.gov/entrez/query/static/clinical.shtml.

7.4.4   Other Considerations

Some other considerations to improve your search include:

- Identifying some possible synonyms for the terms you are searching for. For example, 'prenatal' is a precise medical term that describes things that happen during a pregnancy.
- Using variants of the words. For example, a search on 'pregnancy OR pregnancies' might produce a bigger and better list.
- Don't forget that many words are spelled differently in British English compared to American English (paediatric versus pediatric).
- Use the asterisk, a wild card symbol, to allow for word variants. For example, random* will find random, randomly, randomised, and randomized.

The considerations apply to other systems besides PubMed.

7.4.5   Further reading

- **Developing PubMed Search Skills**. Dalhousie University Libraries. Accessed on 2005-04-28. www.library.dal.ca/kellogg/guides/pubmed/INTROFRM.HTM
- **UF HSCL - PubMed Tutorial**. Libraries UoFHSC. Accessed on 2005-04-28. www.library.health.ufl.edu/pubmed/pubmed2/

7.5   Searching the Internet

When you are trying to find information, your first choice should always be the peer-reviewed literature. The peer-review process is not perfect, but it does eliminate a large number of unsupported research claims. The same cannot be said about the Internet. Still, there are times when the Internet can provide fast and accurate answers. For example, if I am looking for a definition of an alternative medicine therapy that is acceptable to the people who practice that therapy, the Internet will link with various organizations that promote this practice. I also find the Internet helpful for tutorials on things like how to use PubMed.

There are a wide range of search engines on the Internet, and although I usually try Google first, I have found other search engines to work just as well.

You should learn a bit about Boolean logic—how to use words like AND, OR, and NOT to refine your search. Here are some brief tutorials:

- library.albany.edu/internet/boolean.html
- www.lib.duke.edu/libguide/adv_searching.htm
- www.searchability.com/boolean.htm

7.5.1   Gauging the quality of Internet resources

Anyone can publish on the Internet, and there is very little if any attempt to monitor for misleading or even fraudulent claims. Most of the people like me who publish information on the Internet do so without any overt bias or ill intentions, but you still need to be cautious. How do you evaluate a website to see if it provides credible and reliable health information?

There are a variety of things that you should look at. Here are some guidelines loosely based on the Health on the Net Foundation's code of conduct at: www.hon.ch/HONcode/Conduct.html

1. Is the advice being offered by a medically trained professional?
2. Is the advice intended to support rather than replace the care you get from your doctor?
3. Is your confidentiality respected?
4. Is the advice backed up by references and hyperlinks to the original sources?
5. Are the claims presented in a fair and balanced manner?
6. Is it obvious who wrote the material?
7. Are commercial sponsors and noncommercial supporters clearly identified?
8. Is the material on the web page developed independently of any advertising or other sources of revenue?

Be especially aware of material presented by professional organizations and advocacy groups. They do offer a lot of valuable and important information, but are unlikely to produce material that discusses limitations, side effects, and other problems.

7.5.2   Google Scholar

The Google website introduced a new feature in 2004 called Google Scholar (scholar.google.com), in response to complaints that the Google search engine did not find a lot of information stored in library databases. The Google Scholar site will focus on scholarly resources that have been through peer review. It is also a nice way to supplement a PubMed search, because Google Scholar includes all of the PubMed files in its search. This allows you to use some advanced search capabilities that Google has developed which may not be easily available in PubMed. Of course, PubMed has certain search features not available in Google Scholar.

Often a paper published in the peer review literature can also be found at other locations, such as the web pages of the authors. Google Scholar will show you all of the locations of an article, and sometimes you can get the full text for free at the author's web pages.

Google Scholar offers a nice feature that allows you to search for papers that cite a classic or seminal reference. I was interested in finding some recent discussion about spectrum bias, the tendency for some research studies to overstate sensitivity and specificity because they fail to include the full spectrum of disease severity. A search on spectrum bias yields a variety of references. Here are the first five:

- Spectrum bias in the evaluation of diagnostic tests: lessons from the rapid dipstick test for... M.S. Lachs, I. Nachamkin, P.H. Edelstein, J. Goldman, A.R. .... —Cited by 57 - Web Search ... Spectrum bias in the evaluation of diagnostic tests: lessons from the rapid dipstick test for urinary tract infection. Lachs, M.S., Nachamkin ... *Ann Intern Med*, 1992 - ncbi.nlm.nih.gov
- Body mass index compared to dual-energy X-ray absorptiometry: evidence for a spectrum bias F. Curtin, A. Morabia, C. Pichard, D.O. Slosman—Cited by 22 - Web Search Click here to read Body mass index compared to dual-energy X-ray absorptiometry: evidence for a spectrum bias. Curtin, F., Morabia, A., Pichard, C., Slosman, D.O. .... *J. Clin Epidemiol*, 1997 - ncbi.nlm.nih.gov
- Spectrum bias or spectrum effect? Subgroup variation in diagnostic test evaluation S.A. Mulherin, W.C. Miller—Cited by 14 - Web Search ... ACADEMIA AND CLINIC. Spectrum Bias or Spectrum Effect? Subgroup Variation in Diagnostic Test Evaluation. ... Origins of the Concept of Spectrum Bias. ... *Ann. Intern. Med.*, 2002 - annals.org - annals.org - annals.org - ncbi.nlm.nih.gov—all 5 versions
- The effect of spectrum bias on the utility of magnetic resonance imaging and evoked potentials in ... P.W. O'Connor, C.M. Tansay, A.S. Detsky, A.I. Mushlin, W. .... Cited by 10 - Web Search ... ARTICLES. The effect of spectrum bias on the utility of magnetic resonance imaging and evoked potentials in the diagnosis of suspected multiple sclerosis. ... *Ann. Intern. Med.*, 2004 - neurology.org-neurology.org-ncbi.nlm.nih.gov
- Problems of spectrum and bias in evaluating the efficacy of diagnostic tests D.F. Ransohoff, A.R. Feinstein—Cited by 220 - Web Search Original Article from the *New England Journal of Medicine*—Problems of spectrum and bias in evaluating the efficacy of diagnostic tests. ... *N. Engl. J. Med*, 1978—content.nejm.org-ncbi.nlm.nih.gov

The fifth article is obviously a classic, since it was cited by 220 other papers. If you click on the link text 'Cited by 220' you will get all of these papers.

You can also do a similar thing with web pages. For example, you can find all the pages that link to a key page. For example, I routinely refer to the Skeptic's Dictionary (www.skepdic.com) to find material critical of various alternative medicine therapies. It is an easy way to get a different perspective from all the websites that promote alternative medicine. If you wanted to find additional skeptical resources, you could search for all the web pages that link to skepdic.com. Most search engines will let you do this. In Google, you would just search on 'link: www.skepdic.com'.

7.5.3 Sensitive searches versus specific searches

Whenever you search for information, you have to worry about false positives and false negatives. A false positive is an article that appears on your list but it isn't relevant to what you are looking for. A false negative is an article that does not appear on your list, but that is relevant. There is a cost for both false positives and false negatives and you need to think carefully about which is more of a problem for you.

I often search through PubMed or the Internet for interesting teaching examples. If I miss a good example, that's usually okay because there are plenty of others out there. So I find that false negatives are not a serious concern. False positives, though, are more of a problem because they take a lot of time to sort through.

The people conducting a systematic overview, however, have the opposite problem. They do not want to leave out an important study so they try their hardest to get an all-inclusive list. If that means having to sort through a long list, that's just part of the price of assuring a comprehensive search.

Before you conduct your own search, decide what is most important to you. If false positives are the more serious concern, strive for a narrow, specific search. Put in a lot of qualifiers and limitations, and make sure you use 'AND' a lot. This helps ensure that you get a short list that is easy to work through. If false negatives are the more serious concern, then strive for a broad, specific search. Be loose with your search limits and include a wide range of synonyms connected by 'OR'.

7.5.4 Other tips

- Using quote marks to search for an exact phrase leads to a more specific search.
- Restricting your attention to only the most recently published papers might also improve specificity.
- If you find an author who has written one very good and helpful paper, improve your sensitivity by looking for other papers by that same author.
- Once you find a good quality reference, PubMed has a 'Related Articles' link and Google has a 'Similar pages' link that allow you to broaden your search in that particular direction.

7.6 Summary—Where is the evidence?

Write out what you are looking for in the PICO format (Patient, Intervention, Comparison, Outcome). Search for high level sources first and only rely on

PubMed or the Internet if those searches come up empty. Start your PubMed search using single terms that represent broad categories. If these single terms do not yield thousands of hits by themselves, see if another closely related term works better. Use tags and filters in PubMed to narrow your search. Be sure to assess the quality of any source you find on the Internet.

7.7 On your own

1. You have a teenager who is trying to quit smoking and you want to see how group therapy might help compared to a nicotine replacement therapy like a patch or nasal spray. Write out a well focused question using the PICO format.

2. I recently attended a seminar on Reiki therapy. To prepare for the meeting, I wanted to see if there was any published evidence about whether this therapy works. Search for any peer-review articles about Reiki. Try first to find a systematic overview or meta-analysis. If you cannot find such an article, try to find a randomized trial.

3. Repeat this process using Therapeutic Touch.

4. Starting in late 2004, a widely publicized series of randomized trials showed that certain drugs known as Cox-2 inhibitors had an increased risk of cardiac side effects. Was there any published data before 2004 that might suggest that these drugs had an increased risk? Write out an inquiry using the PICO format and search on PubMed for any random-ized clinical trials on Cox-2 inhibitors that might answer this question.

5. Perform a web search on the phrase 'Reiki Therapy' or 'Cognitive Behavioral Therapy' and examine the first ten sites that appear. How many of these pages meet the standards of the HON Code? How far down in the search list do you have to go before you find a source about Reiki therapy that you feel is fair and balanced?

Bibliography

Abramson, J. H. (1990). 'Meta-analysis: A Review of Pros and Cons', *Public Health Reviews*, 18(1): 1–47.

Ackermann-Liebrich, U., Voegeli, T., Gunter-Witt, K., Kunz, I., Zullig, M., Schindler, C., Maurer, M., and Team Z. S. (1996). 'Home Versus Hospital Deliveries: Follow-up Study of Matched Pairs for Procedures and Outcome', *British Medical Journal*, 13(7068): 1313–18. The full text is available at: www.bmj.com/cgi/content/full/313/7068/1313.

Adi, Y., Bayliss, S., Rouse, A., and Taylor, R. S. (2004). 'The Association between Air Travel and Deep Vein Thrombosis: Systematic Review and Meta-analysis', *BMC Cardiovascular Disorders*, 4(1): 7. The full text is available at: www.biomedcentral.com/1471-2261/4/7.

Adkinson, N. F., Jr., Eggleston, P. A., Eney, D., Goldstein, E. O., Schuberth, K. C., Bacon, J. R., Hamilton, R. G., Weiss, M. E., Arshad, H., Meinert, C. L., Tonascia, J., and Wheeler, B. (1997). 'A Controlled Trial of Immunotherapy for Asthma in Allergic Children', *New England Journal of Medicine*, 336(5): 324–31. The full text is available at: www.content. nejm.org/cgi/content/full/336/5/324.

Anderson, H. R., Ayres, J. G., Sturdy, P. M., Bland, J. M., Butland, B. K., Peckitt, C., Taylor, J. C., and Victor, C. R. (2005). 'Bronchodilator Treatment and Deaths from Asthma: Case-Control Study', *British Medical Journal*, 330(7483): 117. The full text is available at: www.pubmedcentral.nih.gov/articlerender.fcgi?tool=pubmed&pubmedid=15618231.

Angell, M. and Kassirer, J. P. (1996). 'Editorials and Conflicts of Interest', *New England Journal of Medicine*, 335(14): 1055–56. The full text is available at: www.content.nejm. org/cgi/content/full/335/14/1055.

Antes, G. and Chalmers, I. (2003). 'Under-reporting of Clinical Trials is Unethical', *Lancet*, 361(9362): 978–9. The full text is available at: www.thelancet.com/journal/vol361/ iss9362/full/llan.361.9362.editorial_and_review.25037.1.

Baer, H. J., Colditz, G. A., Rosner, B., Michels, K. B., Rich-Edwards, J. W., Hunter, D. J., and Willett, W. C. (2005). 'Body Fatness During Childhood and Adolescence and Incidence of Breast Cancer in Premenopausal Women: A Prospective Cohort Study', *Breast Cancer Research*, 7(3): R314–R325. The full text is available at: www.breast-cancer-research. com/content/7/3/R314.

Baker, S. G., Kramer, B. S., and Prorok, P. C. (2004). 'Comparing Breast Cancer Mortality Rates Before-and-After a Change in Availability of Screening in Different Regions: Extension of the Paired Availability Design', *BMC Medical Research Methodology*, 4(1): 12. The full text is available at: www.pubmedcentral.nih.gov/articlerender.fcgi?tool=pubmed& pubmedid=15149551.

Baker, S. G., Lindeman, K. S., and Kramer, B. S. (2001). 'The Paired Availability Design for Historical Controls', *BMC Medical Research Methodology*, 1(1): 9. The full text is available at: www.biomedcentral.com/1471-2288/1/9.

Barnes, D. E. and Bero, L. A. (1998). 'Why Review Articles on the Health Effects of Passive Smoking Reach Different Conclusions', *Journal of the American Medical Association*, 279(19): 1566–70.

Batty, D. (1998). 'Are Sex and Death Related? Study Failed to Adjust for an Important Confounder [letter; comment]', *British Medical Journal*, 316(7145): 1671; discussion 1672. The full text is available at: www.bmj.com/cgi/content/full/316/7145/1671/a.

Bayer, A. and Tadd, W. (2000). 'Unjustified Exclusion of Elderly People from Studies Submitted to Research Ethics Committee for Approval: Descriptive Study', *British Medical Journal*, 321(7267): 992–3. The full text is available at: www.bmj.com/cgi/content/full/321/7267/992.

Bellemare, S., Hartling, L., Wiebe, N., Russell, K., Craig, W.R., McConnell, D., and Klassen, T. P. (2004). 'Oral Rehydration Versus Intravenous Therapy for Treating Dehydration Due to Gastroenteritis in Children: A Meta-analysis of Randomised Controlled Trials', *BMC Medicine*, 2(1): 11. The full text is available at: www.biomedcentral.com/1741–7015/2/11.

Berlin, J. A. (1997). 'Does Blinding of Readers Affect the Results of Meta-analyses?', *Lancet*, 350(9072): 185–6.

Berman, N. G. and Parker, R. A. (2002). 'Meta-analysis: Neither Quick Nor Easy', *BMC Medical Research Methodology*, 2(1): 10. The full text is available at: www.biomedcentral.com/1471-2288/2/10.

Beyerstein, B. L. (1997). 'Why Bogus Therapies Seem to Work', *Skeptical Inquirer*, 21(5). The full text is available at: www.csicop.org/si/9709/beyer.html.

Bhopal, R. (1997). 'Is Research into Ethnicity and Health Racist, Unsound, or Important Science?', *British Medical Journal*, 314(7096): 1751–6. The full text is available at: www.bmj.bmjjournals.com/cgi/content/full/314/7096/1751.

Boden, W. E. (1992). 'Meta-analysis in Clinical Trials Reporting: Has a Tool Become a Weapon?', *American Journal of Cardiology*, 69(6): 681–6.

Booth, I. (2001). 'Does the Duration of Breast Feeding Matter?', *British Medical Journal*, 322(7287): 625–6. The full text is available at: www.bmj.bmjjournals.com/cgi/content/full/322/7287/ 625.

Boyd, E. A., Cho, M. K., and Bero, L. A. (2003). 'Financial Conflict-of-Interest Policies in Clinical Research: Issues for Clinical Investigators', *Academic Medicine*, 78(8): 769–74. The full text is available at: www.academicmedicine.org/cgi/content/full/78/ 8/769.

Brown, J., Kreiger, N., Darlington, G. A., and Sloan, M. (2001). 'Misclassification of Exposure: Coffee as a Surrogate for Caffeine Intake', *American Journal of Epidemiology*, 153(8): 815–20.

Brown, P. J., Warmington, V., Laurence, M., and Prevost, A. T. (2003). 'Randomised Crossover Trial Comparing the Performance of Clinical Terms Version 3 and Read Codes 5 Byte Set Coding Schemes in General Practice', *British Medical Journal*, 326(7399): 1127. The full text is available at: www.bmj.com/cgi/content/full/326/7399/1127.

Bryant, H. E., Visser, N., and Love, E. J. (1989). 'Records, Recall Loss, and Recall Bias in Pregnancy: A Comparison of Interview and Medical Records Data of Pregnant and Postnatal Women', *American Journal of Public Health*, 79(1): 78–80.

Busse, J. W., Bhandari, M., Kulkarni, A. V., and Tunks, E. (2002). 'The Effect of Low-Intensity Pulsed Ultrasound Therapy on Time to Fracture Healing: A Meta-analysis', *Canadian Medical Association Journal*, 166(4): 437–41. The full text is available at: www.cmaj.ca/cgi/content/full/166/4/437.

Buyse, M., Thirion, P., Carlson, R. W., Burzykowski T., Molenberghs, G., and Piedbois, P. (2000). 'Relation Between Tumour Response to First-line Chemotherapy and Survival in Advanced Colorectal Cancer: A Meta-analysis, Meta-Analysis Group in Cancer', *Lancet*, 356(9227): 373–8.

Cameron, E. and Pauling, L. (1976). 'Supplemental Ascorbate in the Supportive Treatment of Cancer: Prolongation of Survival Times in Terminal Human Cancer', *Proceedings of the National Acadamy of Sciences of the United States of America*, 73(10): 3685–9. The full text is available at: www.pubmedcentral.nih.gov/picrender.fcgi?artid= 431183&blobtype=pdf.

Cappelleri, J. C., Ioannidis, J. P., Schmid, C. H., de Ferranti, S. D., Aubert, M., Chalmers, T. C., and Lau, J. (1996). 'Large Trials vs Meta-analysis of Smaller Trials: How do their Results Compare?', *Journal of the American Medical Association*, 276(16): 1332–8.

Carlsen, E., Giwercman, A., Keiding, N., and Skakkebaek, N. E. (1992). 'Evidence for Decreasing Quality of Semen During Past 50 Years', *British Medical Journal*, 305(6854): 609–13.

Carson, P., Ziesche, S., Johnson, G., and Cohn, J. N. (1999). 'Racial Differences in Response to Therapy for Heart Failure: Analysis of The Vasodilator-Heart Failure Trials, Vasodilator-Heart Failure Trial Study Group', *Journal of Cardiac Failure*, 5(3): 178–87.

Cates, C. (2000). 'Lung Cancer and Passive Smoking: Scales for Visual Test of Publication Bias are Unfair', *British Medical Journal*, 321(7270): 1222–3. The full text is available at: www.bmj.bmjjournals.com/cgi/content/full/321/7270/1221.

Chalmers, I. (1990). 'Underreporting Research is Scientific Misconduct', *Journal of the American Medical Association*, 263(10): 1405–8.

Chalmers, T. C. (1991). 'Problems Induced by Meta-analyses', *Statistics in Medicine*, 10(6): 971–9; discussion 979–80.

Chan Carusone, S., Smieja, M., Molly, W., Goldsmih, C. H., Mahoney, J., Chernesky, M., Gnarpe, J., Standish, T., Smith, S., and Loeb, M. (2004). 'Lack of Association Between Vascular Dementia and Chlamydua Pneumoniae Infection: A Case-Control Study', *BMC Neurology*, 4(1): 15. The full text is available at: www.pubmedcentral.nih.gov/articlerender.fcgi?tool= pubmed&pubmedid=15476562.

Chan, K. B., Man-Son-Hing, M., Molnar, F. J., and Laupacis, A. (2001). 'How Well is the Clinical Importance of Study Results Reported? An Assessment of Randomized Controlled Trials', *Canadian Medical Association Journal*, 165(9): 1197–202. The full text is available at: www.cmaj.ca/cgi/content/full/165/9/1197.

Chen, C. L., Gilbert, T. J., and Daling, J. R. (1999). 'Maternal Smoking and Down Syndrome: The Confounding Effect of Maternal Age', *American Journal of Epidemiology*, 149(5): 442–6.

Chen, S., Kumar, S., Chou, W. H., Barrett, J. S., and Wedlund, P. J. (1997). 'A Genetic Bias in Clinical Trials? Cytochrome P450-2D6 (CYP2D6) Genotype in General vs Selected Healthy Subject Populations [letter]', *British Journal of Clinical Pharmacology*, 44(3): 303–4.

Clark, L. C., Combs, G. F., Jr., Turnbull, B. W., Slate, E. H., Chalker, D. K., Chow, J., Davis, L. S., Glover, R. A., Graham, G. F., Gross, E. G., Krongrad, A., Lesher, J. L., Jr., Park, H. K., Sanders, B. B., Jr., Smith, C. L., and Taylor, J. R. (1996). 'Effects of Selenium Supplementation for Cancer Prevention in Patients with Carcinoma of the Skin: A Randomized Controlled Trial'. Nutritional Prevention of Cancer Study Group. *Journal of the American Medical Association*, 276(24): 1957–63.

Colditz, G., Miller, J., and Mosteller, F. (1989). 'How Study Design Affects Outcomes in Comparisons of Therapy I: Medical', *Statistics in Medicine* 8(4): 441–54.

Concato, J., Shah, N., and Horwitz, R. I. (2000). 'Randomized, Controlled Trials, Observational Studies, and the Hierarchy of Research Designs', *New England Journal of Medicine*, 342(25): 1887–92. The full text is available at: www.content.nejm.org/cgi/content/full/342/25/1887.

Cook, D., Guyatt, G., Ryan, G., Clifton, J., Buckingham, L., Willan, A., McIlroy, W., and Oxman, A. (1993). 'Should Unpublished Data be Included in Meta-analyses? Current Convictions and Controversies', *Journal of the American Medical Association*, 269(21): 2749–53.

Cooper, N. J., Sutton, A. J., Abrams, K. R., Wailoo, A., Turner, D., and Nicholson, K. G. (2003). 'Effectiveness of Neuraminidase Inhibitors in Treatment and Prevention of Influenza A & B: Systenatic Review and Meta-Analyses of Randomised Controlled Trials', *British Medical Journal*, 326(7401): 1235. The full text is available at: www.bmj.bmjjournals.com/cgi/content/full/326/7401/1235.

Copas, J. B. (2000). 'Reanalysis of Epidemiological Evidence on Lung Cancer and Passive Smoking', *British Medical Journal*, 320(7232): 417–18.

Corley D. A, Cello, J. P., Adkisson, W., Ko, W. F., and Kerlikowske, K. (2001). 'Octreotide for Acute Esophageal Variceal Bleeding: A Meta-analysis', *Gastroenterology*, 120(4): 946–54. The full text is available at: www.2.us.elsevierhealth.com/scripts/om.dll/serve?retrieve=/pii/S0016508501496739&nav=full.

Cutler, J. A., Grandits, G. A., Grimm, R. H., Thomas, H. E., Billings, J. H., and Wright, N. H. (1991). 'Risk Factor Changes after Cessation of Intervention in the Multiple Risk Factor Intervention Trial', *Preventive Medicine*, 20(2): 183–96.

Danesh, J., Youngman, L., Clark, S., Parish, S., Peto, R., and Collins, R. (1999). 'Helicobacter Pylori Infection and Early Onset Myocardial Infarction: Case-control and Sibling Pairs Study', *British Medical Journal*, 319(7218): 1157–62. The full text is available at: www.bmj.bmjjournals.com/cgi/content/full/319/7218/1157.

Davey Smith, G., Frankel, S., and Yarnell, J. (1997). 'Sex and Death: Are They Related?'. Findings from the Caerphilly Cohort Study. *British Medical Journal*, 315(7123): 1641–4. The full text is available at: www.bmj.bmjjournals.com/cgi/content/full/315/7123/1641.

Davidoff, F., DeAngelis, C., Drazen, J., Hoey, J., Hojgaard, L., Horton, R., Kotzin, S., Nicholls, M., and Nylenna, M. (2001). 'Sponsorship, Authorship and Accountability', *Medical Journal of Australia* 175(6): 294–96. The full text is available at: www.mja. com.au/public/issues/175_06_170901/icmje/icmje.html.

de Torres, J. P., Pinto-Plata, V., Ingenito, E., Bagley, P., Gray, A., Berger, R., and Celli, B. (2002). 'Power of Outcome Measurements to Detect Clinically Significant Changes in Pulmonary Rehabilitation of Patients with COPD', *Chest*, 121(4): 1092–8. The full text is available at: www.chestjournal.org/cgi/content/full/121/4/1092.

de Winter, A. F., Heemskerk, M. A., Terwee, C. B., Jans, M. P., Deville, W., van Schaardenburg, D. J., Scholten, R. J., and Bouter, L. M. (204). 'Inter-observer Reproducibility of Measurements of Range of Motion in Patients with Shoulder Pain Using a Digital Inclinometer', *BMC Musculoskeletal Disorders*, 5(1): 18. The full text is available at: www.biomedcentral.com/1471-2474/5/18.

Deeks, J. J. (2001). 'Systematic Reviews in Health Care: Systematic Reviews of Evaluations of Diagnostic and Screening Tests', *British Medical Journal*, 323(7305): 157–62. The full text is available at: www.bmj.bmjjournals.com/cgi/content/full/323/7305/157.

Derry, S. and Loke, Y. K. (2000). 'Risk of Gastrointestinal Haemorrhage with Long Term Use of Aspirin: Meta-analysis', *British Medical Journal*, 321(7270): 1183–7. The full text is available at: www.bmj.com/cgi/content/full/321/7270/1183.

Des Jarlais, D. C., Paone, D., Milliken, J., Turner, C. F., Miller, H., Gribble, J., Shi, Q., Hagan, H., and Friedman, S. R. (1999). 'Audio-Computer Interviewing to Measure Risk Behaviour for HIV Among Injecting Drug Users: A Quasi-Randomised Trial', *Lancet*, 353(9165): 1657–61.

Devereaux, P. J., Manns, B. J., Ghali, W. A., Quan, H., Lacchetti, C., Montori, V. M., Bhandari, M., and Guyatt, G. H. (2001). 'Physician Interpretations and Textbook Definitions of Blinding Terminology in Randomized Controlled Trials', *Journal of the American Association*, 285(15): 2000–3. The full text is available at: www.jama.ama-assn.org/cgi/content/full/285/15/2000.

Deville, W. L., Buntinx, F., Bouter, L. M., Montori, V. M., De Vet, H. C., Van Der Windt, D. A., and Bezemer P. (2002). 'Conducting Systematic Reviews of Diagnostic Studies: Diadactic Guidelines', *BMC Medical Research Methodology*, 2(1):9. The full text is available at:www.biomedcentral.com/1471-2288/2/9.

Dickersin, K. (1990). 'The Existence of Publication Bias and Risk Factors for its Occurrence', *Journal of the American Medical Association*, 263(10): 1385–9.

Egger, M. and Smith, G. D. (1998). 'Bias in Location and Selection of Studies', *British Medical Journal*, 316(7124): 61–6. The full text is available at: www.bmj.bmjjournals. com/cgi/content/full/316/7124/61.

——Schneider, M., and Davey Smith, G. (1998). 'Spurious Precision? Meta-analysis of Observational Studies', *British Medical Journal*, 316(7125): 140–4. The full text is available at: www.bmj.com/cgi/content/full/316/7125/140.

Elliott, P., Briggs, D., Morris, S., de Hoogh, C., Hurt, C., Jensen, T. K., Maitland, I., Richardson, S., Wakefield, J., and Jarup, L. (2001). 'Risk of Adverse Birth Outcomes in Populations Living Near Landfill Sites', *British Medical Journal*, 323(7309): 363–8. The full text is available at: www.bmj.bmjjournals.com/cgi/content/full/323/7309/363.

Eskenazi, B., Harley, K., Bradman, A., Weltzien, E., Jewell, N. P., Barr, D. B., Furlong, C. E., and Holland, N. T. (2004). 'Association of In Utero Organophosphate Pesticide Exposure and Fetal Growth and Length of Gestation in an Agricultural Population', *Environmental Health Perspectives*, 112(10): 1116–24. The full text is available at: www.ehp.niehs.nih. gov/members/2004/6789/6789.html.

Etminan, M., Gill, S., and Samii, A. (2003). 'Effect of Non-steroidal Anti-inflammatory Drugs on Risk of Alzheimer's Disease: Systematic Review and Meta-analysis of Observational Studies', *British Medical Journal*, 327(7407): 128. The full text is available at: www.bmj.com/cgi/content/full/327/7407/128.

Evans, M. (2000). 'Justified Deception? The Single Blind Placebo in Drug Research', *Journal of Medical Ethics*, 26(3): 188–93. The full text is available at: www.jme.bmjjournals.com/ cgi/content/full/26/3/188.

Eysenck, H. (1978). 'An Exercise in Mega-silliness', *American Psychologist*, 33: 517.

Feinstein, A. R. (1995). 'Meta-analysis: Statistical Alchemy for the 21st Century', *Journal of Clinical Epidemiology*, 48(1): 71–9.

Feise, R. J. (2002). 'Do Multiple Outcome Measures Require p-value Adjustment?', *BMC Medical Research Methodology*, 2(1): 8. The full text is available at: www.biomedcentral.com/1471-2288/2/8.

Fine, L. G., Keogh, B. E., Cretin, S., Orlando, M., and Gould, M. M. (2003). 'How to Evaluate and Improve the Quality and Credibility of an Outcomes Database: Validation and Feedback Study on the UK Cardiac Surgery Experience', *British Medical Journal*, 326(7379): 25–28. The full text is available at: www.bmj.com/cgi/content/full/326/ 7379/25.

Fisch, H. and Goluboff, E. T. (1996). 'Geographic Variations in Sperm Counts: A Potential Cause of Bias in Studies of Semen Quality', *Fertility and Sterility*, 65(5): 1044–6.

Freed, C. R., Greene, P. E., Breeze, R. E., Wei-Yann, T., DuMouchel, W., Kao, R., Dillon, S., Winfield, H., Culver, S., Trojanowski, J. Q., Eidelberg, D., and Fhan, S. (2001). 'Transplantation of Embryonic Dopamine Neurons for Severe Parkinson's Disease', *New England Journal of Medicine*, 344(10): 710–19. The full text is available at: www. content.nejm.org/cgi/content/full/344/10/710.

Gail, M. H. (1996). 'Statistics in Action', *Journal of the American Statistical Association*, 91(433): 1–13.

Geddes, J., Freemantle, N., Harrison, P., and Bebbington, P. (2000). 'Atypical Antipsychotics in the Treatment of Schizophrenia: Systematic Overview and Metaregression Analysis', *British Medical Journal*, 321(7273): 1371–76. The full text is available at: www.bmj. com/cgi/content/full/321/7273/1371.

Glantz, S. A. (2000). 'Lung Cancer and Passive Smoking: Nothing New was Said', *British Medical Journal*, 321(7270): 1222; author reply 1222–3. The full text is available at: www.bmj.bmjjournals.com/cgi/content/full/321/7270/1221.

Glasziou, P., Guyatt, G. H., Dans, A. L., Dans, L. F., Straus, S., and Sackett, D. L. (1998). 'Applying the results of Trials and Systematic Reviews to Individual Patients', *ACP Journal Club*, 129(3): A15–6.

Godwin, M., Ruhland, L., Casson, I., MacDonald, S., Delva, D., Birtwhistle, R., Lam, M., and Seguin, R. (2003). 'Pragmatic Controlled Clinical Trials in Primary Care: The Struggle

Between External and Internal Validity', *BMC Medical Research Methodology*, 3(1): 28. The full text reference is available at: www.biomedcentral.com/1471-2288/3/28.

Goldman, R. D., Macpherson, A., Schuh, S., Mulligan, C., and Pirie, J. (2005). 'Patients Who Leave the Pediatric Emergency Department Without Being Seen: A Case-Control Study', *Canadian Medical Association Journal*, 172(1): 39–43. The full text is available at: www.pubmedcentral.nih.gov/articlerender.fcgi?tool= pubmed&pubmedid=15632403.

Goodwin, R. D. and Pine, D. S. (2002). 'Respiratory Disease and Panic Attacks Among Adults in the United States', *Chest*, 122(2): 645–50. The full text is available at: www.chestjournal.org/cgi/content/full/122/2/645.

Gotzsche, P. C. (1987). 'Reference Bias in Reports of Drug Trials', *British Medical Journal (Clin Res. Ed.)*, 295(6599): 654–6.

——Hammarquist, C., and Burr, M. (1998). 'House Dust Mite Control Measures in the Management of Asthma: Meta-analysis', *British Medical Journal*, 317(7166) 1105–10. The full text is available at: www.bmj.com/cgi/content/full/317/7166/1105.

Gregoire, G., Derderian, F., and Le Lorier, J. (1995). 'Selecting the Language of the Publications Included in a Meta-analysis: Is there a Tower of Babel bias?', *Journal of Clinical Epidemiology*, 48(1): 159–63.

Greenland, S. and O'Rourke, K. (2001). 'On the Bias Produced by Quality Scores in Meta-analysis, and a Hierarchical View of Proposed Solutions', Biostatistics, 2(4): 463–71.

Grimes, D. A. and Schulz, K. F. (2002). 'Bias and Causal Associations in Observational Research', *Lancet*, 359(9302): 248–52. The full text is available at: www.pebita.ch/downloadSTROBE/Grimes-Lancet-2002-Bias.pdf.

Guevara, J. P., Wolf, F. M., Grum, C. M., and Clark, N. M. (2003). 'Effects of Educational Interventions for Self Management of Asthma in Children and Adolescents: Systematic Review and Meta-analysis', *British Medical Journal*, 326(7402): 1308–9. The full text is available at: www.bmj.bmjjournals.com/cgi/content/full/326/7402/1308.

Gunnell, D., Magnusson, P. K., and Rasmussen, F. (2005). 'Low Intelligence Test Scores in 18 Year oldMen and Risk of Suicide: Cohort Study', *British Medical Journal*, 330(7484): 167. The full text is available at: www.pubmedcentral.nih.gov/articlerender.fcgi?tool=pubmed&pubmedid=15615767.

Gustavsson, J. P., Asberg, M., and Schalling, D. (1997). 'The Healthy Control Subject in Psychiatric Research: Impulsiveness and Volunteer Bias', *Acta Psychiatrica Scandinavica*, 96(5): 325–8.

Guyatt, G. H., Juniper, E., Walter, S., Griffith, L, and Goldstein, R. (1998). 'Interpreting Treatment Effects in Randomised Trials', *British Medical Journal*, 316(7132): 690–93. The full text is available at:www.bmj.bmjjournals.com/cgi/content/full/316/7132/690.

Hackshaw, A., Law, M., and Wald, N. (2000). 'Lung Cancer and Passive Smoking: Increased Risk is not Disputed', *British Medical Journal*, 321(7270): 1221–2; author reply 1222–3. The full text is available at:www.bmj.bmjjournals.com/cgi/content/full/321/7270/1221.

Hampel, F., M. D., Ratner, P., M. D., Mansfield, L., M. D., Meeves, S., Pharm, D., Liao, Y., and Georges, G. M. (2003). 'Fexofenadine Hydrochlorida, 180 mg, Exhibits Equivalent Efficacy to Cetirizine, 10 mg, with less Drowsiness in Patients with Moderate-to-Severe Seasonal Allergic Rhinitis', *Annals of Allergy, Asthma, & Immunology*, 91: 354–61, 324–25.

Hansell, A., Hollowell, J., McNiece, R., Nichols, T., and Strachan, D. (2003). 'Validity and Interpretation of Mortality, Health Service and Survey Data on COPD and Asthma in England', *European Respiratory Journal*, 21(2): 279–86. The full text is available at: www.erj.ersjournals.com/cgi/content/full/21/2/279.

Hassan, M. A. and Killick, S. R. (2003). 'Effect of Male Age on Fertility: Evidence for the Decline in Male Fertility with Increasing Age', *Fertility & Sterility*, 79(Suppl 3): 2–9.

Hawkey, C. J. (2001). 'Journals Should See Original Protocols for Clinical Trials', *British Medical Journal*, 323(7324): 1309-. The full text is available at: www.bmj.com/cgi/content/full/323/7324/1309.

Henderson, J., North, K., Griffiths, M., Harvey, I., and Golding, J. (1999). 'Pertussis Vaccination and Wheezing Illnesses in Young Children: Prospective Cohort Study', *British*

Medical Journal, 318(7192): 1173–76. The full text is available at: www.bmj.com/cgi/content/full/318/7192/1173.

Henquet, C., Krabbendam, L., Spauwen, J., Kaplan, C., Lieb, R., and Wittchen Hu, J. O. (2005). 'Prospective Cohort Study of Cannabis Use, Predisposition for Psychosis and Psychotic Symptoms in Young People', *British Medical Journal*, 330(7481): 11. The full text is available at: www.bmj.bmjjournals.com/cgi/content/full/330/7481/11.

Hill, A. B. (1965). 'The Environment and Disease: Association or Causation?', *Proceedings of the Royal Society of Medicine*, 58: 295.

Hollis, S. and Campbell, F. (1999). 'What is Meant by Intention to Treat Analysis? Survey of Published Randomised Controlled Trials', *British Medical Journal*, 319(7211): 670–74. The full text is available at: www.bmj.bmjjournals.com/cgi/content/full/319/7211/670.

Holman, R., Glas, C. A, Lindeboom, R., Zwinderman, A. H., and de Haan, R. J. (2004). 'Practical Methods for Dealing with "not applicable" Item Responses in the AMC Linear Disability Score Project', *Health Qual Life Outcomes*, 2(1): 29. The full text is available at: www.hqlo.com/content/2/1/29.

Homnick, D. N., Anderson, K., and Marks, J. H. (1998). 'Comparison of the Flutter Device to Standard Chest Physiotherapyu in Hospitalized Patients with Cystic Fibrosis: A Pilot Study', *Chest*, 114(4): 993–7. The full text is available at: www.chestjournal.org/cgi/reprint/114/4/993.

Horwitz, R. I. (1987). 'Complexity and Contradiction in Clinical Trial Research', *American Journal of Medicine*, 82(3): 498–510.

—— and Yu, E. C. (1984). 'Assessing the Reliability of Epidemiologic Data Obtained from Medical Records', *Journal of Chronic Diseases*, 37(11): 825–31.

—— Viscoli, C. M., Berkman, L., Donaldson, R. M., Horwitz, S. M., Murray, C. J., Ransohoff, D. F., and Sindelar, J. (1990). 'Treatment Adherence and Risk of Death After a Myocardial Infarction', *Lancet*, 336(8714): 542–5.

Howitt, A. and Armstrong, D. (1999). 'Implementing Evidence Based Medicine in General Practice: Audit and Qualitative Study of Antithrombotic Treatment for Atrial Fibrillation', *British Medical Journal*, 318(7194): 1324–27. The full text is available at www.bmj.bmjjournals.com/cgi/content/full/318/7194/1324.

Hrobjartsson, A. and Gotzsche, P. C. (2001). 'Is the Placebo Powerless? An analysis of Clinical TrialsComparing Placebo with no Treatment', *New England Journal of Medicine*, 344(21): 1594–602. The full text is available at: www.content.nejm.org/cgi/content/full/344/21/1594.

Hsu, L. M. (1989). 'Random Sampling, Randomization, and Equivalence of Contrasted Groups in Psychotherapy Outcome Research', *Journal of Consulting and Clinical Psychology*, 57(1): 131–7.

Hughes, J. R., Giovino, G. A., Klevens, R. M., and Fiore, M. C. (1997). 'Assessing the Generalizability of Smoking Studies', *Addiction*, 92(4): 469–72.

Humphreys, B. K., Delahaye, M., and Peterson, C. K. (2004). 'An Investigation into the Validity of Cervical Spine Motion Palpation Using Subjects with Congenital Block Vertebrae as a "gold standard"', *BMC Musculoskeletal Disorders*, 5(1): 19. The full text is available at: www.biomedcentral.com/1471-2474/5/19.

Humphreys, J. S., Jones, M. P., Jones, J. A., and Mara, P. R. (2002). 'Workforce Retention in Rural and Remote Australia: Determining the Factors that Influence Length of Practice', *Medical Journal of Australia*, 176(10): 472–6. The full text is available at: www.mja.com.au/public/issues/176_10_200502/hum10169_fm.html.

Hunter, P. R., Bickerstaff, K., and Davies, M. A. (2004). 'Potential Sources of Bias in the Use of Individual's Recall of the Frequency of Exposure to Air Pollution for Use in Exposure Assessment in Epidemiological Studies: A Cross-sectional Survey', *Environmental Health*, 3(1): 3. The full text is available at: www.ehjournal.net/content/3/1/3.

Husereau, D., Shukla, V., Boucher, M., Mensinkai, S., and Dales, R. (2004). 'Long Acting Beta2 Agonists for Stable Chronic Obstructive Pulmonary Disease with Poor Reversibility: A Systematic Review of Randomised Controlled Trials', *BMC Pulmonary Medicine* 4(1): 7. The full text is available at: www.biomedcentral.com/1471-2466/4/7.

Hussain, A. and Smith, R. (2001). 'Declaring Financial Competing Interests: Survey of Five General Medical Journals', *British Medical Journal*, 323(7307): 263–4. The full text is available at: www.bmj.com/cgi/content/full/323/7307/263.

Jacobs, J., Jimenez, L. M., Gloyd, S. S., Gale, J. L., and Crothers, D. (1994). 'Treatment of Acute Childhood Diarrhea with Homeopathic Medicine: A Randomized Clinical Trial in Nicaragua', *Pediatrics*, 93(5): 719–25.

Jadad, A., Moore, A., Carroll, D., Jenkinson, C., Reynolds, D., Gavaghan, D., and McQuay, H. (1996). 'Assessing the Quality of Reports of Randomized Controlled Trials: Is Blinding Necessary?', *Controlled Clinical Trials*, 17(1): 1–12.

Jain, A., Concato, J., and Leventhal, J. M. (2002). 'How Good Is the Evidence Linking Breastfeedingand Intelligence?', *Pediatrics*, 109(6): 1044–53. The full text is available at: www.pediatrics.aappublications.org/cgi/content/full/109/6/1044.

Johnson, A. G. and Dixon, J. M. (1997). 'Removing Bias in Surgical Trials', *British Medical Journal*, 314(7085): 916–7. The full text is available at: www.bmj.bmjjournals.com/cgi/content/full/314/7085/916.

Johnson, L. R., Doherty, G., Lairmore, T., Moley, J. F., Brunt, L. M., Koenig, J., and Scott, M. G. (2001). 'Evaluation of the Performance and Clinical Impact of a Rapid Intraoperative Parathyroid Hormone Assay in Conjunction with Preoperative Imaging and Concise Parathyroidectomy', *Clinical Chemistry*, 47(5): 919–25. The full text is available at: www.clinchem.org/cgi/content/full/47/5/919.

Jordan, R., Gold, L., Cummins, C., and Hyde, C. (2002). 'Systematic Review and Metaanalysis of Evidence for Increasing Numbers of Drugs in Antiretroviral Combination Therapy', *British Medical Journal*, 324(7340): 757. The full text is available at: www.bmj.com/cgi/content/full/324/7340/757.

Jorm, A. F., Kitchener, B. A., O'Kearney, R., and Dear, K. B. (2004). 'Mental Health First Aid Training of the Public in a Rural Area: A Cluster Randomized Trial [ISRCTN53887541]', *BMC Psychiatry*, 4(1): 33. The full text is available at: www.biomedcentral.com/1471-244X/4/33.

Juni, P., Altman, D. G., and Egger, M. (2001). 'Systematic Reviews in Health Care: Assessing the Quality of Controlled Clinical Trials', *British Medical Journal*, 323(7303): 42–6. The full text is available at: www.bmj.com/cgi/content/full/323/7303/42.

Kaasinen, V., Nurmi, E., Bergman, J., Eskola, O., Solin, O., Sonninen, P., and Rinne, J. O. (2001). 'Personality Traits and Brain Dopaminergic Function in Parkinson's Disease', *Proceedings of the National Academy of Sciences of the United States of America*, 98(23): 13272–7. The full text is available at: www.pnas.org/cgi/content/full/98/23/13272.

Karvonen, M., Cepaitis, Z., and Tuomilehto, J. (1999). 'Association Between Type 1 Diabetes and Haemophilus Influenzae Type b Vaccination: Birth Cohort Study', *British Medical Journal*, 318(7192): 1169–72. The full text is available at: www.bmj.bmjjournals.com/cgi/content/full/318/7192/1169.

Kennedy, A. D., Leigh-Brown, A. P., Torgerson, D., Campbell, J. H., and Grant, A. (2002). 'Resource Use Data By Patient Report or Hospital Records: Do They Agree?', *BMC Health Services Research*, 2(1): 2. The full text is available at: www.biomedcentral.com/1472-6963/2/2.

Kimmel, S. E., Berlin, J. A., Reilly, M., Jaskowiak, J., Kishel, L., Chittams, J., and, Strom, B.L. (2005). 'Patients exposed to rofecoxib and celecoxib have different odds of nonfatal myocardial infarction',. *Annals of Internal Medicine*, 142(3) 157–64. The full text is available at: http://www.acponline.org/journals/annals/myo_infar.pdf.

Kinnunen, T. I., Luoto, R., Gissler, M., Hemminki, E., and Hilakivi-Clarke, L. (2004). 'Pregnancy Weight Gain and Breast Cancer Risk', *BioMed Central*, 4(1): 7. The full text is available at: www.pubmedcentral.nih.gov/articlerender.fcgi?tool=pubmed&pubmedid =15498103.

Kjaergard, L. and Gluud, C. (2002). 'Citation Bias of Hepato-Biliary Randomized Clinical Trials', *Journal of Clinical Epidemiology*, 55(4): 407–10.

Kjaergard, L. L., Villumsen, J., and Gluud, C. (2001). 'Reported Methodologic Quality and Discrepancies Between Large and Small Randomized Trials in Meta-analyses', *Annals of Internal Medicine*, 135(11): 982–9. The full text is available at: www.annals.org/cgi/ reprint/135/11/982.pdf.

Kliethermes, P., Cross, M., Lanese, M., Johnson, K., and Simon, S. (1999). 'Transitioning Preterm Infants with Nasogastric Tube Supplementation: Increased Likelihood of Breast-feeding', *Journal of Obstetric, Gynecologic, and Neonatal Nursing*, 28(3): 264–73.

Koch, A., Hörmann, A., Löwel, H., and Senges, J. (1997). Published in the Proceedings of the International Conference on Nonrandomized Comparative Clinical Studies in Heidelberg, April 10–11. '"The 60-Minutes-Myocardial Infarction Project": Comparison with a Registry and a Randomized Clinical Trial'. Accessed on 2003-06-30. www.symposion. com/nrccs/koch.htm

Kramer, M.S., Guo, T., Platt, R. W., Shapiro, S., Collet, J. P., Chalmers, B., Hodnett, E., Sevkovskaya, Z., Dzikovich, I., and Vanilovich, I. (2002). 'Breastfeeding and Infant Growth: Biology or Bias?', *Pediatrics*, 110(2 Pt 1): 343–7. The full text is available at: www.pediatrics.aappublications.org/cgi/reprint/110/2/343.

Kulkarni, M., Elsner, C., Ouellet, D., and Zeldin, R. (1994). 'Heparinized Saline Versus Normal Saline in Maintaining Patency of the Radial Artery Catheter', *Canadian Journal of Surgery*, 37(1): 37–42.

Lachs, M. S., Nachamkin, I., Edelstein, P. H., Goldman, J., Feinstein, A. R., and Schwartz, J. S. (1992). 'Spectrum Bias in the Evaluation of Diagnostic Tests: Lessons from the Rapid Dipstick Test for Urinary Tract Infection', *Annals of Internal Medicine*, 117(2): 135–40.

Lakits, A., Prokesch, R., Bankier, A., Weninger, F., and Imhof, H. (1998). 'Multiplanar Imaging in the Preoperative Assessment of Metallic Intraocular Foreign Bodies. Helical Computed Tomography Versus Conventional Computed Tomography', *Ophthalmology*, 105(9): 1679–85.

Lampe, J. W. (1999). 'Health Effects of Vegetables and Fruit: Assessing Mechanisms of Action of Human Experimental Studies', *American Journal of Clinical Nutrition*, 70(3 Suppl): 475S–490S. The full text is available at: www.ajcn.org/cgi/content/full/70/3/475S.

Law, M. R., Wald, N. J., and Rudnicka, A. R. (2003). 'Quantifying Effect of Statins on Low Density Lipoprotein Cholesterol, Ischaemic Heart Disease, and Stroke: Systematic Review and Meta-analysis', *British Medical Journal*, 326(7404): 1423. The full text is available at: www.bmj.bmjjournals.com/cgi/content/full/326/7404/1423.

Lawlor, D. A. and Hopker, S. W. (2001). 'The Effectiveness of Exercise as an Intervention in the Management of Depression: Systematic Review and Meta-regression Analysis of Randomised Controlled Trials', *British Medical Journal*, 322(7289): 763. The full text is available at: www.bmj.com/cgi/content/full/322/7289/763.

Lazarou, J., Pomeranz, B. H., and Corey, P. N. (1998). 'Incidence of Adverse Drug Reactions in Hospitalized Patients: A Meta-analysis of Prospective Studies', *Journal of the American Medical Association*, 279(15): 1200–5.

Le, G. M., O'Malley, C. D., Glaser, S. L., Lynch, C. F., Stanford, J. L., Keegan, T. H. M., and West, D. W. (2004). 'Breast Implants Following Mastectomy in Women with Early-Stage Breast Cancer: Prevalence and Impact on Survival', *Breast Cancer Research*, 7(2): R184–R193. The full text is available at: www.breast-cancer-research.com/content/7/2/ r184.

Lee, S., Walker, J. R., Jakul, L., and Sexton, K. (2004). 'Does Elimination of Placebo Responders in a Placebo Run-In Increase the Treatment in Randomized Clinical Trials? A Meta-Analytic Evaluation', *Depression and Anxiety*, 19(1): 10–9.

Lesson, C. P., Kattenhorn, M., Deanfield, J. E., and Lucas, A. (2001). 'Duration of Breast Feeding and Arterial Distensibility in Early Adult Life: Population Based Study', *British Medical Journal*, 322(7287); 643–7. The full text is available at: www.bmj.com/cgi/content/full/322/7287/643.

Lefering, R. and Neugebauer, E. (1997). Published in the Proceedings of the International Conference on Nonrandomized Comparative Clinical Studies in Heidelberg, April 10–11. Problems of Randomized Controlled Trails (RCT) in Surgery. Accessed on 2003-06-30. www.symposion.com/nrccs/lefering.htm.

Leibovici, L. (2001). 'Effects of Remote, Retroactive Intercessory Prayer on Outcomes in Patients with Bloodstream Infection: Randomised Controlled Trial', *British Medical Journal*, 323(7327): 1450–1. The full text is available at: www.bmj.bmjjournals.com/cgi/content/full/323/7327/1450.

LeLorier, J., Gregoire, G., Benhaddad, A., Lapierre, J., and Derderian, F. (1997). 'Discrepancies Between Meta-Analyses and Subsequent Large Randomized, Controlled Trials', *New England Journal of Medicine*, 337(8): 536–42. The full text is available at: www.content.nejm.org/cgi/content/full/337/8/536.

Leuchter, A. F., Cook, I. A., Witte, E. A., Morgan, M., and Abrams, M. (2002). 'Changes in Brain Function of Depressed Subjects During Treatment With Placebo', *American Journal of Psychiatry*, 159(1): 122–9. The full text is available at: www.ajp.psychiatryonline.org/cgi/reprint/159/1/122.

Lexchin, J., Bero, L. A., Djulbegovic, B., and Clark, O. (2003). 'Pharmaceutical Industry Sponsorship and Research Outcome and Quality: Systematic Review', *British Medical Journal*, 326(7400): 1167–70. The full text is available at: www.bmj.com/cgi/content/full/326/7400/1167.

Liberati, A., Himel, H. N., and Chalmers, T. C. (1986). 'A Quality Assessment of Randomized Control Trials of Primary Treatment of Breast Cancer', *Journal of Clinical Oncology*, 4(6): 942–51.

Lichtenstein, D. R., and Wolfe, M. M. (2000). 'COX-2-Selective NSAIDs: New and Improved', *Journal of the American Medical Association*, 284(10): 1297–9.

Lilienfeld, S. O., Wood, J. M., and Garb, H. N. (2001). 'What's Wrong with This Picture?', *Scientific American*, 284(5) 80–7. A pdf version of this paper is available at: www.psychologicalscience.org/pdfreq.cfm? PATH_INFO=/newsresearch/publications/journals/sa1_2.pdf& VARACTION=GO&CFID=1205220&CFTOKEN=17007476.

Liu, J., Kjaergard, L. L., and Gluud, C. (2002). 'Misuse of Randomization: A Review of Chinese Randomized Trials of Herbal Medicines for Chronic Hepatitis B', *American Journal of Chinese Medicine*, 30(1): 173–6.

Logar, C. M., Pappas, L. M., Ramkumar, N., and Beddhu, S. (2005). 'Surgical Revascularization Versus Amputation for Peripheral Vascular Disease in Dialysis Patients: A Cohort Study', *BMC*, 6(1): 3. The full text is available at: www.biomedcentral.com/1471-2369/6/3.

Lucassen, P. L., Assendelft, W. J., Gubbels, J. W., van Eijk, J. T., van Geldrop, W. J., and Neven, A. K. (1998). 'Effectiveness of Treatments for Infantile Colic: Systematic Review', *British Medical Journal* 316(7144): 1563–9. The full text is available at: www.bmj.com/cgi/content/full/316/7144/1563.

Ludbrook, J. (2003). 'Interim Analyses of Data as They Accumulate in Laboratory Experimentation', *BMC Medical Research Methodology*, 3(1): 15. The full text is available at: www.biomedcentral.com/1471-2288/3/15.

Lumley, J., Oliver, S., and Waters, E. (2000). 'Interventions for Promoting Smoking Cessation During Pregnancy', *Cochrane Database of Systematic Reviews*, (2) CD001055.

Macleod, J., Davey Smith, G., Heslop, P., Metcalfe, C., Carroll, D., and Hart, C. (2002). 'Psychological Stress and Cardiovascular Disease: Empirical Demonstration of Bias in a Prospective Observational Study of Scottish Men', *British Medical Journal*, 324(7348): 1247–51. The full text is available at: www.bmj.bmjjournals.com/cgi/content/full/324/7348/1247.

Maher, C. G., Sherrington, C., Herbert, R. D., Moseley, A. M., and Elkins, M. (2003). 'Reliability of the PEDro Scale for Rating Quality of Randomized Controlled Trials', *Physical Therapy*, 83(8): 713–21.

Mahoney, M. C., Bauer, J. E., Tumiel, L., McMullen, S., Schieder, J., and Pikuzinski, D. (2002). 'Longitudinal Impact of a Youth Tobacco Education Program', *BMC Family Practice*, 3(1): 3. The full text is available at: www.biomedcentral.com/1471-2296/3/3.

Malcoe, L. H., Duran, B. M., and Montgomery, J. M. (2004). 'Socioeconomic Disparities in Intimate Partner Violence Against Native American Women: A Cross-sectional Study', *BMC Med*, 2(1): 20. The full text is available at: www.biomedcentral.com/1741-7015/2/20.

Mallinckrodt, C. H., Raskin, J., Wohlreich, M. M., Watkin, J. G., and Detke, M. J. (2004). 'The Efficacy of Duloxetine: A Comprehensive Summary of Results From MMRM and LOCF_ANCOVA in Eight Clinical Trials', *BMC Psychiatry*, 4(1): 26. The full text reference is available at: www.biomedcentral.com/1471-244x/4/26.

Mandelblatt, J. S., Kanetsky, P., Eggert, L., and Gold, K. (1999). 'Is HIV Infection a Co-factor for Cervical Squamous Cell Neoplasia?', *Cancer Epidemilogy, Biomarkers & Prevention*, 8(1): 97–106. The full text is available at: www.cebp.aacrjournals.org/cgi/content/full/8/1/97.

Mann, C. J. (2003). 'Observational Research Methods. Research Design II: Cohort, Cross Sectional, and Case-control Studies', *Emergency Medicine Journal*, 20(1): 54–60. The full text is available at: www.emj.bmjjournals.com/cgi/content/full/20/1/54.

Mann, H. (2002). 'Research Ethics Committees and Public Dissemination of Clinical Trial Results', *Lancet*, 360(9330): 406.

Mann, J. (2002). 'Truths About the NINDS Study: Setting the Record Straight', *Western Journal of Medicine*, 176(3): 192–4. The full text is available at: www.ewjm.com/cgi/content/full/176/3/192.

Marsh, J. L., Hutton, J. L., and Binks, K. (2002). 'Removal of Radiation Dose Response Effects: An Example of Over-Matching', *British Medical Journal*, 325(7359): 327–30. The full text is available at: www.bmj.bmjjournals.com/cgi/content/full/325/7359/327.

Martin, G. S., Eaton, S., Mealer, M., and Moss, M. (2005). 'Extravascular Lung Water in Patients with Severe Sepsis: A Prospective Cohort Study', *Critical Care Medicine*, 9(2): R74–R82. The full text is available at: www.ccforum.com/content/9/2/r74.

Mason, L., Moore, R. A., Edwards, J. E., Derry, S., and McQuay, H. J. (2004). 'Topical NSAIDs for Chronic Musculoskeletal Pain: Systematic Review and Meta-analysis', *BMC Musculoskeletal Disorders*, 5(1): 28. The full text is available at: www.biomedcentral.com/1471-2474/5/28.

Mayor, S. (2001). 'Row Over Breast Cancer Screening Shows that Scientists Bring Some Subjectivity Into Their Work', *British Medical Journal*, 323(7319): 956. The full text is available at: http://bmj.com/cgi/content/full/323/7319/956.

Maziak, W., Ward, K. D., Rastam, S., Mzayek, F., and Eissenberg, T. (2005). 'Extent of Exposure to Environmental Tobacco Smoke (ETS) and its Dose-Response Relation toRespiratory Health Among Adults', *Respiratory Research*, 6(1): 13. The full text is available at: http://respiratory-research.com/content/6/1/13.

McAlister, F. A., O'Connor, A. M., Wells, G. A., Fgrover, S. A., and Laupacis, A. (2000). When Should Hypertension Be Treated? The Different Perspectives of Canadian Family Physicians and Patients', *Canadian Medical Association Journal*, 163(4): 403–8. The full text is available at: www.cmaj.ca/cgi/content/full/163/4/403.

McNamee, R. and Dolk, H. (2001). 'Does Exposure to Landfill Waste Harm the Fetus? Perhaps, but More Evidence is Needed', *British Medical Journal*, 323(7309): 351–2. The full text is available at: bmj.bmjjournals.com/cgi/content/full/323/7309/351.

Meade, T. W. and Brennan, P. J. (2000). 'Determination of Who May Derive Most Benefit from Aspirin in Primary Prevention: Subgroup Results from a Randomised Controlled Trial', *British Medical Journal*, 321(7252): 13–17. The full text is available at: bmj.bmjjournals.com/cgi/content/full/321/7252/13.

Meinert, C. L. and Gilpin, A. K. (2001). 'Estimation of Gender Bias in Clinical Trials', *Statistics in Medicine*, 20(8): 1153–64.

Moertel, C., Fleming, T. R., Creagan, E. T., Rubin, J., O'Connell, M. J., and Ames, M. M. (1985). 'High-dose Vitamin C Versus Placebo in the Treatment of Patients with Advanced Cancer Who Have Had No Prior Chemotherapy: A Randomized Double-blind Comparison', *New England Journal of Medicine*, 312(3): 137–41.

Moinpour, C. M., Lyons, B., Schmidt, S. P., Chansky, K., and Patchell, R. A. (2000). 'Substituting Proxy Ratings for Patient Ratings in Cancer Clinical Trials: An Analysis Based on a Southwest Oncology Group Trial in Patients with Brain Metastases', *Quality of Life Research*, 9(2): 219–31.

Mortensen, E. M., Cornell, J., and Whittle, J. (2004). 'Racial Variations in Processes of Care for Patients with Community-Acquired Pneumonia', *BMC Health Services Research*, 4(20): The full text is available at: www.biomedcentral.com/1472-6963/4/20.

National Emphysema Treatment Trial Research Group (2001). 'Patients at High Risk of Death After Lung-volume-reduction Surgery', *New England Journal of Medicine*, 345(15): 1075–83. A pdf version of this paper is available at: www.content.nejm.org/cgi/reprint/345/15/1075.pdf.

Nelemans, P. J., Rampen, F. H., Ruiter, D. J., and Verbeek, A. L. (1995). 'An Addition to the Controversy on Sunlight Exposure and Melanoma Risk: A Meta-analytical Approach', *Journal of Clinical Epidemiology*, 48(11): 1331–42.

Nelson, M. (1986). 'The Distribution of Nutrient Intake Within Families', *British Journal of Nutrition*, 55(2): 267–77.

Noseworthy, J. H., Ebers, G. C., Vandervoort, M. K., Farquhar, R. E., Yetisir, E., and Roberts, R. (1994). 'The Impact of Blinding on the Results of a Randomized, Placebo-controlled Multiple Sclerosis Clinical Trial', *Neurology*, 44(1): 16–20.

Ola, B., Papaioannou, S., Afnan, M. A., Hammadieh, N., and Gimba, S. (2001). 'Recombinant or Urinary Follicle-stimulating Hormone? A Cost-effectiveness Analysis Derived by Particularizing the Number Needed to Treat from a Published Meta-analysis', *Fertil Steril*, 75(6): 1106–10.

Olsen, G. W., Bodner, K. M., Ramlow, J. M., Ross, C. E., and Lipshultz, L. I. (1995). 'Have Sperm Counts Been Reduced 50 Percent in 50 Years? A Statistical Model Revisited', *Fertility and Sterility*, 63(4): 887–93.

Olsen, O. and Gotzsche, P. C. (2001). 'Screening for Breast Cancer with Mammography', *CochraneDatabase of Systematic Reviews*, (4): CD001877.

Olshansky, B. and Dossey, L. (2003). 'Retroactive Prayer: A Preposterous Hypothesis?', *British Medical Journal*, 327(7429): 1465–8. The full text is available at: www.bmj.bmjjournals.com/cgi/content/full/327/7429/1465.

Park, R. L. (1997). 'Alternative Medicine and the Laws of Physics', *Skeptical Inquirer*, 21(5): 24–8. The full free text of this reference is available at: www.csicop.org/si/9709/park.html.

Perneger, T. V. (1988). 'What's Wrong with Bonferroni Adjustments', *British Medical Journal*, 316(7139): 1236–8. The full text is available at: www.bmj.com/cgi/content/full/316/7139/1236.

Piland, S. G., Motl, R. W., Ferrara, M. S., and Peterson, C. L. (2003). 'Evidence for the Factorial and Construct Validity of a Self-Report Concussion Symptoms Scale', *Journal of*

Athlete Training, 38(2): 104–12. The full text is available at: www.pubmedcentral.nih.gov/articlerender. fcgi?tool=pubmed&pubmedid=12937520.

Pimlott, H. J., Hux, J. E., Wilson, L. M., Kahan, M., Li, C., and Rosser, W. W. (2003). 'Educating Physicians to Reduce Benzodiazepine Use by Elderly Patients: A Randomized Controlled Trial', *Canadian Medical Association Journal*, 168(7): 835–9. The full text is available at: www.cmaj.ca/cgi/content/full/168/7/835.

Pollex, R., Hegele, B., and Ban, M. R. (2001). 'Research of the Holiday Kind: Celestial Determinants of Success in Research', *Canadian Medical Association Journal*, 165(12): 1584. The full text is available at: www.cmaj.ca/cgi/content/full/165/12/1584.

Portnoy, J. M. and Simon, S. D. (2003). 'Is 3-mm Less Drowsiness Important?', *Annals of Allergy, Asthma and Immunology*, 91(4): 324–25.

Powell, C. V., Kelly, A. M., and Williams, A. (2001). 'Determining the Minimum Clinically Significant Difference in Visual Analog Pain Score for Children', *Annals of Emergency Medicine*, 37(1): 28–31.

Ramasubbu, K., Gurm, H., and Litaker, D. (2001). 'Gender Bias in Clinical Trials: Do Double Standards Still Apply?', *Journal of Women's Health and Gender Based Medicine*, 10(8): 757–64.

Randolph, A. G., Cook, D. J., Gonzales, C. A., and Andrew, M. (1998). 'Benefit of Heparin in Peripheral Venous and Arterial Catheters: Systematic Review and Meta-analysis of Randomised Controlled Trials', *British Medical Journal*, 316(7136): 969–75. The full text is available at: www.bmjjournals.com/cgi/content/full/316/7136/969.

Ransohoff, D. F. and Feinstein, A. R. (1978). 'Problems of Spectrum and Bias in Evaluating the Efficacy of Diagnostic Tests', *New England Journal of Medicine*, 299(17): 926–30.

Ray, W. A., Daugherty, J. R., and Griffin, M. R. (2002). 'Lipid-lowering Agents and the Risk of Hip Fracture in a Medicaid Population', *Injury Prevention*, 8(4): 276–9. The full text is available at: www.ip.bmjjournals.com/cgi/content/full/8/4/276.

Roberts, C. and Torgerson, D. (1999). 'Understanding Controlled Trials: Baseline imbalance in Randomised Controlled Trials', *British Medical Journal*, 319(7203): 185. The full text is available at: www.bmj.com/cgi/content/full/319/7203/185.

Rochon, P. A., Binns, M. A., Litner, J. A., Litner, G. M., Fischbach, M. S., Eisenberg, D., Kaptchuk, T. J., Stason, W. B., and Chalmers, T. C. (1999). 'Are Randomized Control Trial Outcomes Influenced by the Inclusion of a Placebo Group? A Systematic Review of Nonsteroidal Antiinflammatory Drug Trials for Arthritis Treatment', *Journal of Clinical Epidemiology*, 52(2): 113–22.

Ronning, O. M. and Guldvog, B. (1999). 'Should Stroke Victims Routinely Receive Supplemental Oxygen? A Quasi-randomized Controlled Trial', *Stroke*, 30(10): 2033–7. The full text is available at: www.intl-stroke.ahajournals.org/cgi/content/full/30/10/2033.

Rosenbaum, P. R. (1995). Observational Studies. New York NY: Springer Verlag.

Rosenbaum, P. R. (2001). 'Replicating Effects and Biases', *American Statistician*, 55(3): 223–7.

Rothman, K. J. and Greenland, S. (1998). Modern Epidemiology. Philadelphia PA: Lippincott, Williams, and Wilkins.

Sackett, D. L. (1997). 'Evidence-based Medicine and Treatment Choices', *Lancet*, 349(9051): 570; discussion 572–3.

Salas, M., Ward, A., and Caro, J. (2002). 'Are Proton Pump Inhibitors the First Choice for Acute Treatment of Gastric Ulcers? A Meta-analysis of Randomized Clinical Trials', *BMC Gastroenterology*, 2(1): 17. The full text is available at: www.biomedcentral.com/1471-230X/2/17.

Salo, P. M., Xia, J., Johnson, C. A., Li, Y., Kissling, G. E., Avol, E. L., Liu, C., and London, S. J. (2004). 'Respiratory Symptoms in Relation to Residential Coal Burning and Environmental Tobacco Smoke Among Early Adolescents in Wuhan, China: A Cross-sectional Study',

Environmental Health, 3(1): 14. The full text is available at: www.ehjournal.net/content/3/1/14.

Sarasua, S. and Savitz, D. A. (1994). 'Cured and Broiled Meat Consumption in Relation to Childhood Cancer: Denver, Colorado (United States)', *Cancer Causes Control*, 5(2): 141–8.

Schellevis, F. G., van der Velden, J., van de Lisdonk, E., van Eijk, J. T., and van Weel, C. (1993). 'Comorbidity of Chronic Diseases in General Practice', *Journal of Clinical Epidemiology*, 46(5): 469–73.

Schulz, K. F. (1996). 'Randomised Trials, Human Nature, and Reporting Guidelines', *Lancet*, 348(9027): 596–8.

Schulz, K. F., Chalmers, I., and Altman, D. G. (2002). 'The Landscape and Lexicon of Blinding in Randomized Trials', *Annals of Internal Medicine*, 136(3): 254–59. The full text is available at: www.annals.org/cgi/content/full/136/3/254.

—— Chalmers, I., Hayes, R., and Altman, D. (1995). 'Empirical Evidence of Bias Dimensions of Methodological Quality Associated with Estimates of Treatment Effects in Controlled Trials', *Journal of American Medical Association*, 273(5): 408–12.

Schwartz, A. L., Meek, P. M., Nail, L. M., Fargo, J., Lundquist, M., Donofrio, M., Grainger, M., and Throckmorton, T. (2002). 'Mateo M. Measurement of Fatigue Determining Minimally Important Clinical Differences', *Journal of Clinical Epidemiology*, 55(3): 239–44.

Scollo, M., Lal, A., Hyland, A., and Glantz, S. (2003). 'Review of the Quality of Studies on the Economic Effects of Smoke-free Policies on the Hospitality Industry', *BMJ Tobacco Control*, 12(1): 13–20. The full text is available at: www.tc.bmjjournals.com/cgi/content/full/12/1/13.

Sen, A. (2002). 'Health: Perception Versus Observation', *British Medical Journal*, 324(7342): 860–1. The full text is available at: www.bmj.com/cgi/content/full/324/7342/860.

Senn, S. (1997). 'Are Placebo Run Ins Justified?', *British Medical Journal*, 314(7088): 1191–3. The full text is available at: www.bmj.com/cgi/content/full/314/7088/1191.

—— (2002). 'Maintaining the Integrity of the Scientific Record: Scientific Standards Observed by Medical Journals Can Still be Improved', *British Medical Journal*, 324(7330): 169.

Shapiro, S. (1994). 'Meta-analysis/Shmeta-analysis', *American Journal of Epidemiology*, 140(9): 771–8.

Siderowf, A. D. (2004). 'Evidence from Clinical Trials: Can We Do Better?', *Neurorx*, 1(3): 363–71. The full text is available at: www.pubmedcentral.nih.gov/articlerender.fcgi?tool=pubmed&pubmedid=15717039.

Silverstein, F.E., Faich, G., Goldstein, J. L., Simon, L. S., Pincus, T., Whelton, A., Makuch, R., Eisen, G., Agrawal, N. M., Stenson, W. F., Burr, A. M., Zhao, W. W., Kent, J. D., Lefkowith, J. B, Verburg, K. M., and Geis, G. S. (2000). 'Gastrointestinal Toxicity with Celecoxib vs Nonsteroidal Anti-inflammatory Drugs for Osteoarthritis and Rheumatoid Arthritis: The CLASS Study: A Randomized Controlled Trial. Celecoxib Long-term Arthritis Safety Study', *Journal of the American Medical Association*, 284(10): 1247–55.

Smith, T. A., House, R. F., Jr., Croghan, I. T., Gauvin, T. R., Colligan, R. C., Offord, K. P., Gomez-Dahl, L. C., and Hurt, R. D. (1996). 'Nicotine Patch Therapy in Adolescent Smokers', *Pediatrics*, 98(4 Pt 1): 659–67.

Snapinn, S. M. (2000). 'Noninferiority Trials', *Current Control Trials in Cardiovascular Medicine*, 1(1): 19–21. A pdf version of this paper is available at: www.cvm.controlled-trials.com/content/pdf/cvm-1-1-019.pdf.

Sokal, D., Irsula, B., Hays, M., Chen-Mok, M., and Barone, M. A. (2004). 'Vasectomy by Ligation and Excision, With or Without Fascial Interposition: A Randomized Controlled Trial [ISRCTN77781689]', *BMC Medicine*, 2(1): 6. The full text is available at: www.biomedcentral.com/1741-7015/2/6.

Steptoe, A., Doherty, S., Rink, E., Kerry, S., Kendrick, T., and Hilton, S. (1999). 'Behavioural Counselling in General Practice for the Promotion of Healthy Behaviour Among Adults at Increased Risk of Coronary Heart Disease: Randomised Trial', *British Medical Journal*, 319(7215): 943–7; discussion 947–8. The full text is available at: www.bmj.bmjjournals. com/cgi/content/full/319/7215/943.

Stern, J. and Simes, R. (1997). 'Publication Bias: Evidence of Delayed Publication In a Cohort Study of Clinical Research Projects', *British Radical Journal*, 315(7109): 640–5. The full text is available at: www.bmj.bmjjournals.com/cgi/content/full/315/7109/640.

Stocks, N. and Gunnell, D. (2000). 'What Are the Characteristics of General Practitioners Who Routinely Do Not Return Postal Questionnaires: A Cross Sectional Study', *Journal of Epidemiology and Community Health*, 54(12): 940–1. The full text is available at: jech.bmjjournals.com/cgi/reprint/54/12/940.

Strassberg, D. S. and Lowe, K. (1995). 'Volunteer Bias in Sexuality Research', *Archives of Sexual Behaviour*, 24(4): 369–82.

Sutton, A. J., Duval, S. J., Tweedie, R. J., Abrams, K. R., and Jones, D. R. (2000). 'Empirical Assessment of Effect of Publication Bias on Meta-analyses', *British Medical Journal*, 320: 1574–77. The full text is available at: www.bmj.com/cgi/content/full/320/7249/1574.

Swaen, G. G., Teggeler, O., and van Amelsvoort, L. G. (2001). 'False Positive Outcomes and Design Characteristics in Occupational Cancer Epidemiology Studies', *International Journal of Epidemiology*, 30(5): 948–54. The full text is available at: www.ije.oxfordjournals. org/cgi/content/full/30/5/948.

Swaim, R. C., Beauvais, F., Chavez, E., and Oetting, E. (1997). 'The Effect of School Dropout Rates on Estimates of Adolescent Substance Use among Three Racial/Ethnic Groups', *American Journal of Public Health*, 87(1): 51–5.

Tang, J. L., and Liu, J. L. (2000). 'Misleading Funnel Plot for Detection of Bias in Meta-analysis', *Journal of Clinical Epidemiology* 53(5): 477–84.

Tang, J.-L., Zhan, S., and Ernst, E. (1999). 'Review of Randomised Controlled Trials of Traditional Chinese Medicine', *British Medical Journal*, 319(7203): 160–1. The full text is available at: www.bmj.com/cgi/content/full/319/7203/160.

Taylor, A. L., Ziesche, S., Yancy, C., Carson, P., D'Agostino, R. B., Jr., Ferdinand, K., Taylor, M. A., Adams, K., Sabolinski, M., Worcel, M., and Cohn, J. N. (2004). 'Investigators A-AHFT. Combination of Isosorbide dinitrate and Hydralazine in Blacks with Heart Failure', *New England Journal of Medicine*, 351(20): 2049–57. The full text is available at: www.content.nejm.org/cgi/content/full/351/20/2049.

Taylor, R. S., Reeves, B. C., Ewings, P. E., and Taylor, R. J. (2004). 'Critical Appraisal Skills Training for Health Care Professionals: A Randomized Controlled Trial [ISRCTN46272378]', *British Medical Journal of Medical Education*, 4(1): 30. The full text is available at: www.biomedcentral.com/content/pdf/1472-6920-4-30.pdf.

Teekachunhatean, S., Kunanusorn, P., Rojanasthien, N., Sananpanich, K., Pojchamarnwiputh, S., Lhieochaiphunt, S., and Pruksakorn, S. (2004). 'Chinese Herbal Recipe Versus Diclofenac in Symptomatic Treatment of Osteoarthritis of the Knee: A Randomised Controlled Trial [ISRCTN70292892', *British Medical Journal of Complementary and Alternative Medicine*, 4(1): 19. The full text is available at: www.pubmedcentral.nih.gov/articlerender.fcgi?tool= pubmed&pubmedid=15588333.

Thomson, C. E., Crawford, F., and Murray, G. D. (2005). 'The Effectiveness of Extra Corporeal Shock Wave Therapy for Plantar Heel Pain: A Systematic Review and Meta-analysis', *BMC Musculoskeletal Disorders*, 6(1): 19. The full text is available at: www. biomedcentral.com/1471-2474/6/19.

Tonnelier, J-M., Prat, G., Le Gal, G., Gut-Gobert, C., Renault, A., Boles, J.-M., and L'Her, E. (2005). 'Impact of a Nurses' Protocol-Directed Weaning Procedure on Outcomes in Patients Undergoing Mechanical Ventilation for Longer than 48 Hours: A Prospective Cohort

Study with a Matched Historical Control Group', *Critical Care*, 9(2): R83–R89. The full text is available at: www.ccforum.com/content/9/2/r83.

Tramer, M., Reynolds, D., Moore, R., and McQuay, H. (1997). 'Impact of Covert Duplicate Publication on Meta-analysis: A Case Study', *British Medical Journal*, 315(7109): 635–40. The full text is available at: www.bmj.bmjjournals.com/cgi/content/full/315/7109/635.

Tyas, S. L., Manfreda, J., Strain, L. A., and Montgomery, P. R. (2001). 'Risk Factors for Alzheimer's Disease: A Population-Based, Longitudinal Study in Manitoba, Canada', *International Journal of Epidemiology*, 30(3): 598–9. The full text is available at: http://ije.oxfordjournals.org/cgi/content/full/30/3/590.

Vickers, A., Goyal, N., Harland, R., and Rees, R. (1998). 'Do Certain Countries Produce Only Positive Results? A Systematic Review of Controlled Trials', *Controlled Clinical Trials*, 19(2): 159–66.

Wacholder, S. (1995). 'Design Issues In Case-control Studies', *Statistical Methods in Medical Research*, 4(4): 293–309.

Wainer, H. and Brown, L. M. (2004). 'Two Statistical Paradoxes in the Interpretation of Group Differences: Illustrated with Medical School Admission and Licensing data', *The American Statistician*, 58(2): 117–23.

——Pamer, S., and Bradlow, E. T. (1998). 'A Selection of Selection Anomalies', *Chance*, 11(2): 3–7.

Walsh, C. and Ross, L. F. (2003). 'Whether and Why Pediatric Researchers Report Race and Ethnicity', *Archives of Pediatrics & Adolescent Medicine*, 157(7): 671–5.

Weijer, C. (2002). 'I Need a Placebo Like I Need a Hole in the Head', *Journal of Law & Medical Ethics*, 30(1): 69–72.

Wentz, R. (2002). 'Visibility of Research: FUTON Bias', *Lancet*, 360(9341): 1256.

Yoshioka, A. (1998). 'Use of Randomisation in the Medical Research Council's clinical Trial of Streptomycin in Pulmonary Tuberculosis in the 1940's', *British Medical Journal*, 317(7167): 1220–3. The full text is available at: www.bmj.bmjjournals.com/cgi/content/full/317/7167/1220.

Index